THE ULTIMATE SEASONAL LUNCHBOX

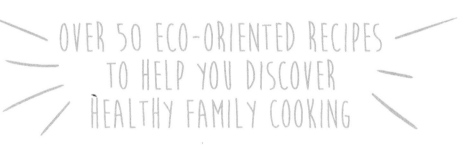

OVER 50 ECO-ORIENTED RECIPES
TO HELP YOU DISCOVER
HEALTHY FAMILY COOKING

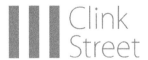

Clink
Street

Published by Clink Street Publishing 2022

Copyright © 2022

First edition.

ISBN:
978-1-914498-84-8 - paperback
978-1-914498-85-5 - ebook

CONTENTS

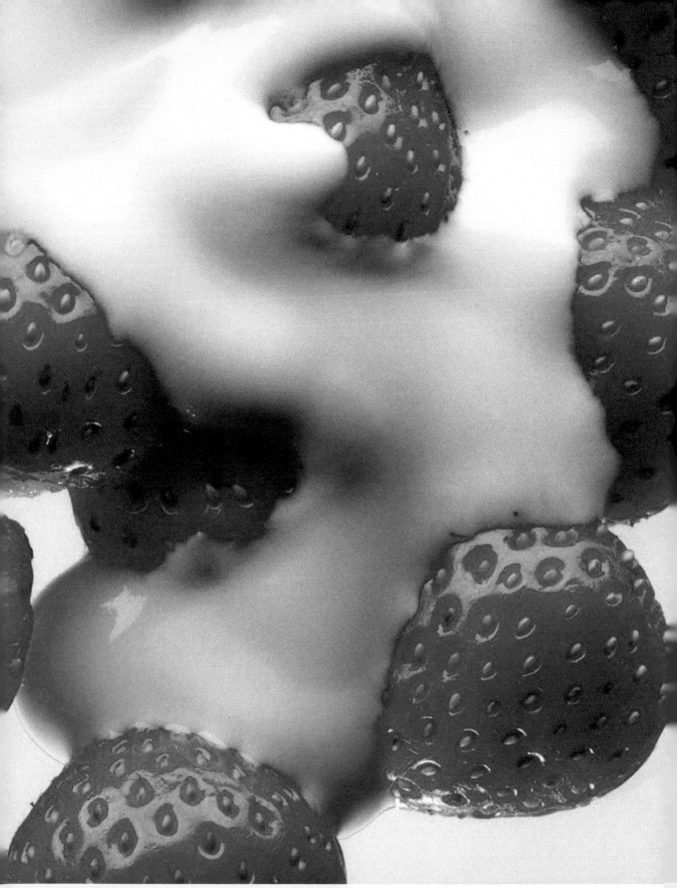

INTRODUCTION

Childhood eating habits can have a huge impact on children's health throughout adolescence and adulthood. Eating food containing important nutrients helps children grow, and is essential for children's mental and physical development.

Introducing a balanced diet does not mean restricting foods or calories. On the contrary, getting a balanced diet signifies eating a wide variety of nutritious foods from all the different food groups including fruit and vegetables, wholegrains such as brown rice, wholegrain bread and wholegrain pasta, beans and lentils, lean meat and fish, seeds and nuts.

The majority of children go through phases with their eating, but their habits also change over time. Something they would have never eaten before will suddenly become a favourite. It is important to expose them to a variety of healthy foods, and to find creative ways of including important nutrients in their daily intake. Disguising vegetables in pasta, soups and patties is a great way to add important nutrients in their foods and to train their palates with new flavours.

A crucial part of a healthy diet is to avoid processed foods because they contain extra fat, salt and sugar to enhance their flavour. This will eventually have a negative impact on children's health by increasing significantly the risk of overweight, obesity, diabetes, high blood pressure, and other health problems in adolescence and adulthood.

Preparation is fundamental when following a healthy lifestyle. Planning meals for the week ahead is a great strategy to save time without compromising taste and a well-balanced diet.

This handy lunchbox guide to family cooking offers useful advice on healthy choices, with numerous ideas that can be prepared in advance for those busy days. It is allergy-friendly and completely free from nuts. Many schools have food policies to reduce the risk of accidental exposure. Parents play an important role by following these policies and packing food products that are safe. The recipes can be easily adapted to gluten and lactose free by replacing ingredients.

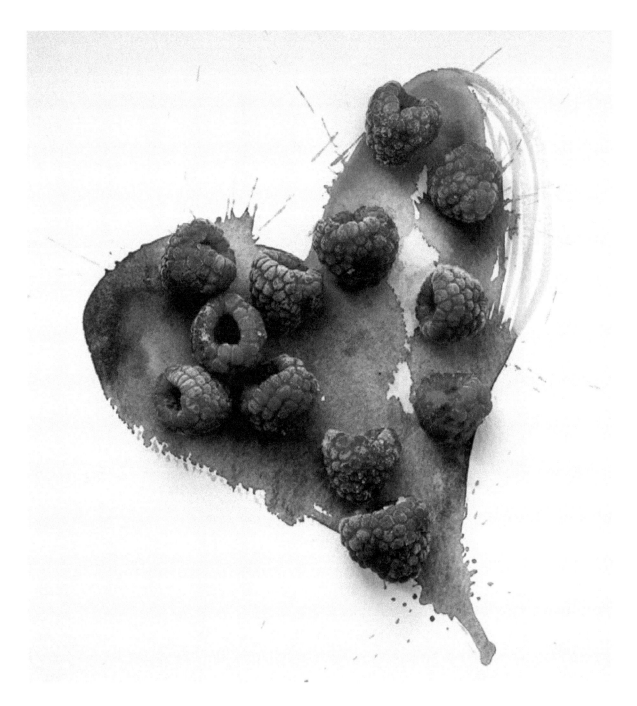

The healthier option is to cook from scratch avoiding processed food, artificial colourings and additives. The lunchboxes are creatively assembled to make the food attractive by combining the different textures and colours of fruit and vegetables because the varied colours contain different nutrients and health benefits.

The preparation process is not complicated, so kids may enjoy preparing their lunches themselves. It is an easy and gradual process and is not very time-consuming. Children can experiment replacing foods and making their own combinations using this book as reference.

Let them choose what they want to eat for their lunches from the groups of food. Children love to be involved in decision-making, and this book is designed to attract their curiosity.

As a parent, I believe in leading by example. Eating healthy foods shows your child how enjoyable a healthy lifestyle can be. The book is planned with parents in mind. Lunchboxes are appetising, delicious and healthy. Parents can easily duplicate them for the whole family.

A HEALTHY LUNCHBOX SETS HABITS THAT HAVE LIFELONG CANCER PREVENTION BENEFITS

When it comes to organising school lunches, it can be a chore trying to arrange everything together for a perfect meal. This book promotes the preparation of different foods for the whole family. The recipes are nutritionally balanced in hope that healthy lunches may be enjoyed every day.

Planning daily school lunches is not only a headache and a time-consuming process but it is easy to run out of ideas after a couple of months. It may seem that repetition cannot be avoided. We have planned out a set of ideas that fit kids' lunchboxes neatly and conveniently for every day. We hope this book will prove a practical solution to busy parents around the world.

The recipes are created for our preferred lunchbox. Bento boxes combinations are endless and have been around for centuries. They are the premier solution to a lunch mess problem because they contain multiple compartments within their own container, designed to separate different foods. They allow you to fit several different types and portions of food, all in one package. Bento lunchboxes also offer an added functionality because food will not jostle together or spill.

The food mentioned in each recipe in this book may be collectively packed in a bento lunchbox or used singularly as a dinner or a single compartment lunchbox.

THE HISTORY AND CULTURE OF BENTO LUNCHBOXES

Bento boxes have existed since the Kamakura period in Japan. During that period, workers who went out in the fields brought with them every day bento boxes packed with both cooked and dried rice known as Hoshi-ii. As time went on, Bento lunchboxes became more refined and common practice, as travellers took bento lunchboxes filled with different kinds of food everywhere with them.

It is easier to get creative when packing a lunch in a bento box. You can arrange different types of food in different ways to really make an appetising lunchbox experience. The best part is that all the different foods will not jumble or mix together thereby ruining the taste, consistence and visual experience of the food.

Lunchboxes come in different shapes and sizes, but they all have one factor in common, namely the practicality and simplicity of compartments which separate different types of foods within the same container.

Whether you want to mix your meat and rice, pasta and vegetables, or separate the two of them or even combine all three food groups, a bento lunchbox allows for any possible combination or separation of food. The portion-controlled compartments that separate foods in the bento lunchbox make it possible to include a variety of healthy food, thereby promoting a healthy diet.

With bento lunchboxes all kinds of meals and snacks may be transported conveniently. They are designed to fit easily into a backpack, briefcase or purse. Food will not fall out. Instead it will stay together though still separate. Packing a bento box for your children to take to school is undoubtedly one of the best decisions a parent can make on a daily basis. Children will learn to love their bento lunchbox and will be excited for lunch every day without the boring monotony and unhealthy nutrition of a daily sandwich.

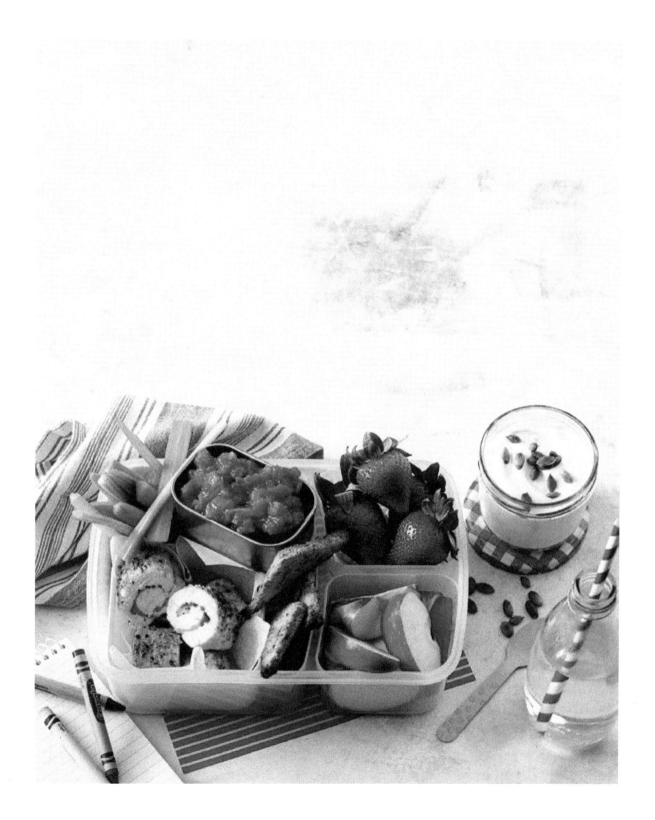

WHAT CHILDREN SHOULD DRINK

Guidelines say that babies need only breast milk or infant formula and, once they are six months old, small amounts of water. Children should stick to milk. water and occasionally fresh fruit juice.

Drinking too many artificial colourings found in soda, fruit juice or any sugary drink is linked to many health complications. Guidelines recommend that children between the age of one and two years should drink two to three cups of whole milk a day. At the age of two and three, they should drink no more than two cups of skimmed or low-fat milk a day. For age four and five, they should drink no more than two and a half cups of skimmed or low-fat milk a day.

With regard to water, it is (i) a half-cup to a cup for six to twelve-month-old children, (ii) one to four cups a day for ages one to three, and (iii) one-and-a-half to five cups a day for four and five-year-olds, adding a cup per year after that.

Diarrhea, constipation, increased upper respiratory infections and skin rashes are signs of a possible cow's milk dairy intolerance. In that case, switching to a dairy-free milk like soy, almond, oat, or coconut milk might be a solution.

WHAT CHILDREN SHOULD HAVE INSTEAD OF COW'S MILK

Plant-based milks, like almond or coconut, are fortified with calcium and vitamin D. However they do not contain nearly the amount of bioavailable protein as dairy cow's milk. Soy milk does compare to cow's milk in terms of protein, and additionally offers a great source of calcium, vitamin D, iron and B-vitamins.

Most cow's milk is fortified with vitamin D, which the body needs in order to absorb calcium. You may also get calcium and vitamin D from whole foods in addition to plant-based milk. Foods containing vitamin D include oily fish such as salmon, sardines, herring and mackerel, and also red meat, liver, egg yolks and fortified foods such as some sandwich spreads and breakfast cereals. Calcium-rich foods include salmon, spinach, cheese, yoghurt and almonds.

Giving your children plant-based milk instead of dairy is perfectly fine, given that they eat enough protein. Soy milk contains the most balanced nutritional profile of the plant milk family and also offers a complete source of protein. Ultimately, incorporating a variety of plant-based milk can ensure proper nutrient delivery and absorption. Choosing unsweetened versions limits added sugars and carrageenan.

Carrageenan is processed powder made from dried seaweed. Compared to fresh, vitamin-packed seaweed, carrageenan has a different chemical structure. It is used as a thickening agent. Products containing carrageenan might include dairy products and dairy substitutes, ice cream, processed meat, frozen pizza and infant formula. Studies have shown that carrageenan may promote inflammation, bloating and irritability in the bowels.

MAKING HEALTHIER CHOICES

Supermarkets are profit driven. The way they operate is by ordering large quantities, pile the stock in their warehouses and sell it cheaply. The main problem with such a system is that products with very long expiration dates actually contain a high amount of additives and preservatives.

As the name suggests, preservatives are used to lengthen the shelf life of food items and also maintain the flavour of food for a long time. Artificial or chemical preservatives that are used to delay the contamination of food are the ones which lead to health problems. These preservatives are artificially produced and are synthetic in nature. They are often labelled as additives on food.

Using considerable amounts of preservatives over the years can have a negative impact on our health. One of the most harmful effects of preservatives in food items is their ability to transform into carcinogen agents. Some of the food items consist of nitrosamine, a preservative which has nitrites and nitrates which mix with gastric acids and form cancer-causing agents as well as heart disease and breathing problems.

Fresh produce is not only packed with more flavour than supermarket food but is also free from harmful additives and preservatives. The fresher the food, the tastier it is. This largely depends on storage time. Food that is stored for long periods loses sugar and starch, and that greatly affects flavour. Taste and texture also depend on where fruit and vegetables are grown and where animals are farmed and live. Greenhouses produce less flavour in some fruit and vegetables than those which are grown on good farmland. Profit-driven fruit and vegetable growers deliberately modify their produce to make it look more appealing, knowing that supermarket shoppers do not taste before they buy.

Livestock that is solely raised outdoors in good conditions produces tastier meat than animals forced to live in barns. The former eat natural, nutritious food. On the contrary, animals forced to live in barns feed on inorganic grains enhanced with growth hormones. Animals which are free to roam about produce more tender and flavoursome meat. This concept applies also to wild fish, in the sense that wild fish has more flavour than farmed fish. This is largely due to diet, fresher water, and seasonality.

It is not just about the flavour. Eating food that is in season has huge health advantages. Choosing ingredients that are naturally in season ensures that one gets fresher, sweeter and perfectly ripe produce that tastes better. This enriches the meals that you prepare and ensures that you do not end up with spoilt, impaired produce that has been kept refrigerated for months while being transported from one country to another.

Besides, seasonal food supports what your body needs. For example, summer foods, such as stone fruits, help protect against sun damage since they are packed with carotenoids.

SEASONAL FOODS AND THE ENVIRONMENT

Seasonal foods are environmentally friendly. Consuming foods that are in season helps the environment in several ways. Most supermarket foods will travel long distances before reaching your shopping basket. The negative impact on the environment is due to the amount of fuel used.

Seasonal produce straight from the field, orchard or the sea dramatically reduces fuel pollution and other harmful chemicals used in the storage and transportation process. Supermarket food packaging burdens the environment by using enormous amounts of energy, thereby damaging chemicals and harmful waste that end up in landfills. Fresh, local produce, on the other hand, has minimal packaging, often with simple paper bag. This not only has less impact on the flavour of the food, but reduces the use of natural resources.

USING GOOD-QUALITY INGREDIENTS

In this book, we are proposing healthier treats by cooking from scratch at home where you can control the ingredients. Ready-made products often contain low-quality ingredients, including cheap processed fats, fake chocolate chips and substance which add shelf life.

When shopping for baking ingredients, look for free-range eggs, organic products and high-quality flour. You may even opt for wholemeal flour, gluten-free flour or chickpea flour.

You need to keep in mind that cookies, loaves and cakes taste really good because they contain a fair amount of sugar and fat. In this publication, we have reduced the excess amounts of fat and sugar, but added other ingredients that are much healthier without compromising the taste of the final product.

Baking home-made cookies, cakes and loaves may be a stress reliever. All the recipes are easy and uncomplicated. They are designed to include the children in the process... a perfect family affair on rainy days.

Overall, if you do not have time to bake everything from scratch, buy the highest-quality products. Avoid ingesting unnecessary additives and preservatives that are harmful to your health. All foods can fit into a healthy diet. It is all about moderation, balance and portion sizes. It is better to vary foods, insert treats and satisfy your cravings rather than eating ten other things which distract you from a cookie.

The key to a balanced diet is quality over quantity, using real butter, vanilla, high cocoa percentage chocolate, good-quality flour and free-range eggs, without adding additives and artificial flavours. Your effort will produce a much healthier option and will taste far superior than ready-made products. Another way to save on fat and sugar is by avoiding toppings. Using such delicious ingredients, toppings may easily be left out without them being missed.

BUTTER VERSUS MARGARINE

Butter has earned a bad reputation for being high in saturated fats. It is about 50% to 60% saturated fat, while margarine is only about 9% saturated. And that is why margarine was introduced as a healthier alternative. Later on, however, researchers, nutritionists and health experts have come to realise that butter is healthier than margarine as the latter is heavily processed from vegetable oil.

Reducing the amount of saturated fats is advisable for a healthy balanced diet. In this recipe book, a minimal amount of butter is used to bake the sweet treats. Reducing spreads and cream, frosting and butter cream in the preparation of bakes and sandwiches reduces the calorie intake without limiting the options to have delicious treats in your lunchbox. Processed foods, artificial colouring and additives have been discarded in the compilation of this book.

THE EASIEST WAY TO PEEL POMEGRANATES

Pomegranates are delicious and good for you. Unfortunately some people are put off by the task of removing the seeds from a pomegranate because they think it is finicky, time-consuming and messy. The easiest way is to pop out the seeds under water. Place a large salad bowl filled with water directly in a sink. Slice off the flowering end of the pomegranate and score the peel in quarters. You do not have to score deeply. Submerge the pomegranate in the bowl of water and gently pry it apart. Keeping it submerged prevents berries and juice from spraying or somehow staining you. While the pomegranate is still under water, use your fingers to wiggle and pry all of the seeds, which are called arils, thereby freeing them from the core of the pomegranate.

Use your hands or a sieve to skim the pith out of the water. The seeds will sink to the bottom of the bowl and the pith will float. Finally, scoop up the arils by the handful and run them under some cold water in order to rinse away any last bits of pith.

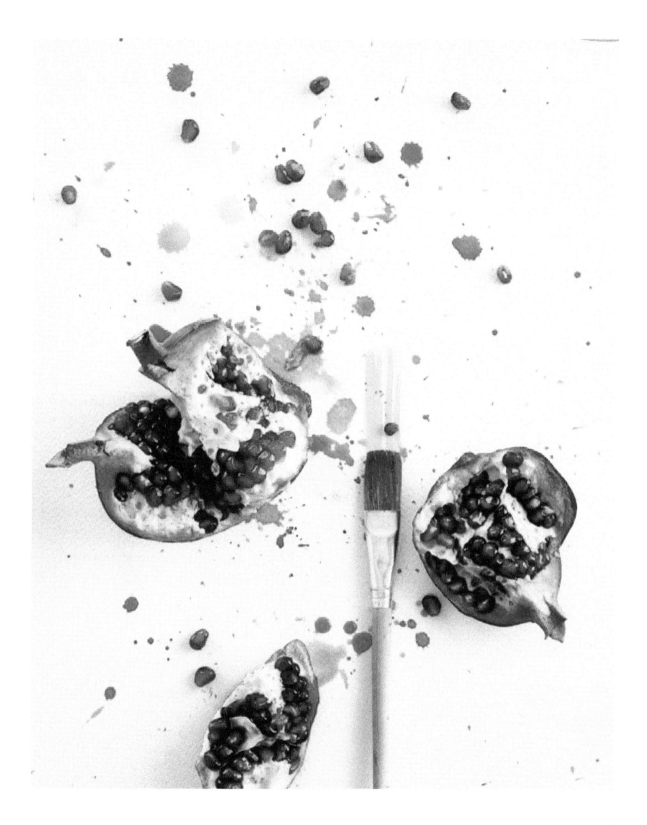

HOW TO SEGMENT AN ORANGE IN SUPREMES

This French technique is a bit more complicated, but the rewards, which are legion, result in tender segments of orange without any of that pesky, chewy membrane.

Stabilise the orange with a very sharp small knife or a flexible fish knife. Slice off both ends of the orange to expose the flesh. Place the orange with one cut end down on the cutting board.

Cut off the peel, working as close to the citrus flesh as possible. Cut along the curve of the fruit to remove a section of peel, thereby exposing the fruit underneath. Once the peel is off, trim any remaining bits of pith which may still be clinging to the orange.

Segment it out, working over a bowl. Hold the peeled and pithless orange in your non-dominant hand and, using a knife, carefully cut along the membranes to slice out each segment. Let the segments fall into the bowl. Continue rotating the fruit and cutting out the supremes until you have separated all of the membranes from the citrus supremes. Use your utility knife to remove any seeds that might still be attached once you remove the membranes. Finally, squeeze the orange core once you have removed the segments. There is plenty of tasty juice still inside.

HOW TO PREVENT CUT APPLES FROM BROWNING

Stir two tablespoons of honey into a cup of water and soak your apple slices in the mixture for 30 seconds. This will avoid your apples from browning because there is a compound in honey that stops the enzyme responsible for oxidation. Additionally, this is one of the methods that will not unpleasantly alter the apple's taste.

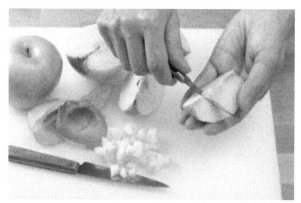
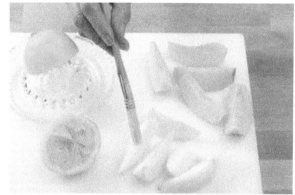
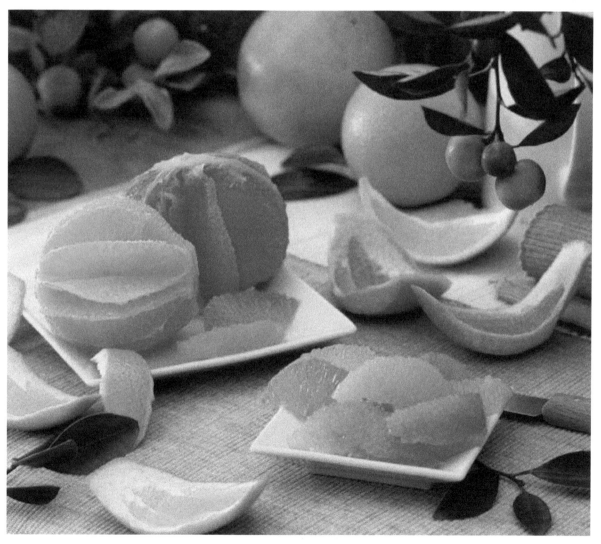

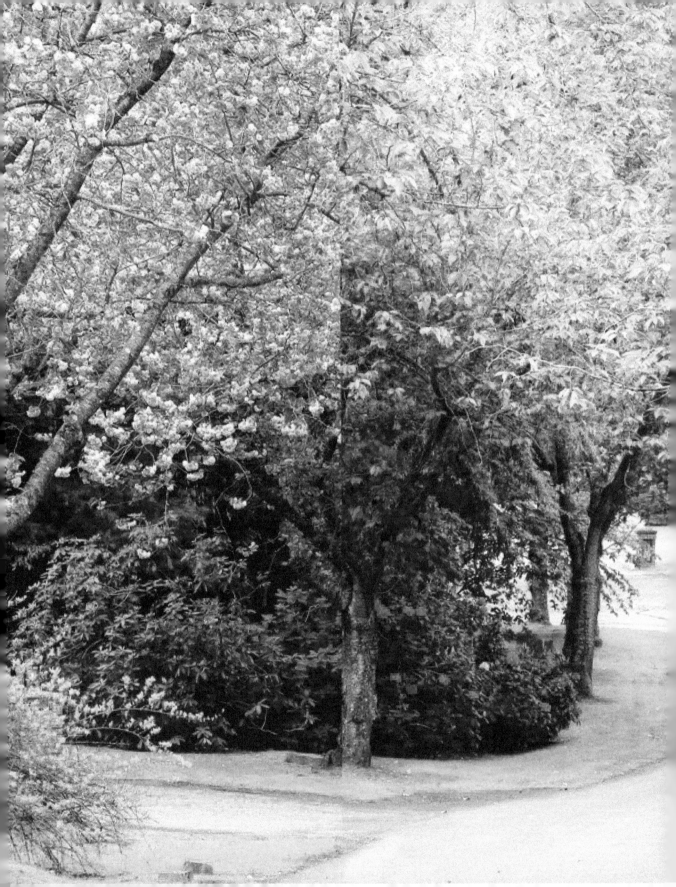

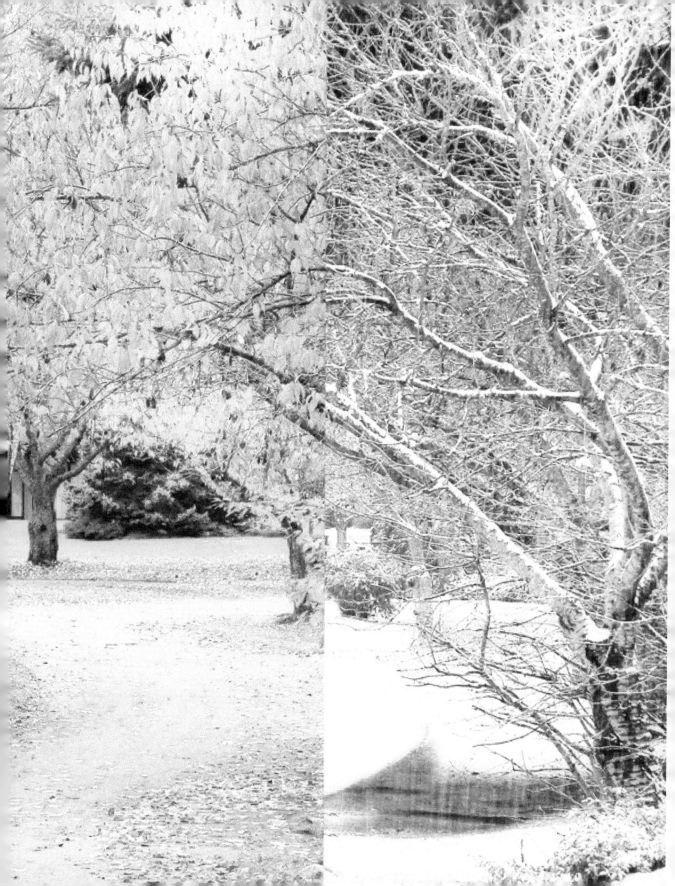

THE FOUR SEASONS

A season is a period of the year that is distinguished by special climate conditions. The four seasons – spring, summer, autumn and winter – follow one another regularly. Each has its own light, temperature, and weather patterns that repeat yearly.

These patterns are an important element in our lives. They influence what we wear, what we eat and what we do in our free time. The seasonal weather, especially rain and sunshine, also affects our mood.

In ancient civilisations, people observed that the sun was at different places during different times of the year. But they failed to understand how this led to the changes in the seasons themselves.

Towards the end of the Middle Ages, the astronomer Copernicus changed one's view of the solar system. He understood that the sun, and not the earth, was at its centre and that objects moved around it. Today we know that earth moves around the sun. This means that the northern and southern parts of the earth get different amounts of sunlight throughout the year. Nowadays, we call these solar patterns seasons.

Seasons play a very important part in agriculture as well. Seasonal fruit and vegetables cannot adjust to any kind of temperature. They are therefore not available all year round, and are grown in a natural cycle of seasons during their suitable climate.

Eating seasonal fruits, vegetables, fish and meat is an important part of a healthy and sustainable diet. These provide essential vitamins, minerals, dietary fibre and proteins. Seasonal produce also has a lower environmental impact because the produce is abundant and controlled during its particular season.

AUTUMN

Autumn is the season that follows summer and foreshadows winter. This season may also be called fall. It is the time when big changes in nature and environment happen.

Animals start their preparation for cold months and plants stop making food. Nature slowly begins to fall asleep. Temperatures become cooler and rainfalls become frequent. Of course, the main sign of autumn is when leaves change their colour and the scenery becomes more dramatic, magnificent and beautiful. Days get shorter and nights longer. The moon is brighter in this period of year and also some new stars may be visible.

Autumn is a meaningful time to enjoy the harvests cultivated earlier in the year. Farmers and gardeners collect apples, pumpkins, pears, corn and other different crops because, should the first frost come suddenly, all efforts made throughout the year would have been in vain.

The changing seasons are key points in the cycle of life in nature, and within this cycle, nutritious produce becomes available for us to eat. The colder air of autumn provides a variety of vibrantly coloured fruit and robust root vegetables including:

APPLES, BANANAS, BEETS, BELL PEPPERS, BROCCOLI, BRUSSELS SPROUTS, CABBAGE, CARROTS, CAULI OWER, CELERY, COLLARD GREENS, CRANBERRIES, GARLIC, GINGER, GRAPES, GREEN BEANS, KIWI-FRUIT, LEMONS, LETTUCE, LIMES, MANGOS, MUSHROOMS, ONIONS, PARSNIPS, PEARS, PEAS, PINEAPPLES, POTATOES, PUMPKIN, RADISHES, RASPBERRIES, SPINACH, SWEET POTATOES, SWISS CHARD, TURNIPS

MUSHROOMS

Mushrooms are fungi, and they grow differently from fruits and vegetables. Mushrooms are decomposers and break down dead plants to recycle their nutrients. Even though they are almost entirely water, they are a great source of vitamin B, selenium and potassium.

A fun fact about mushrooms is that they have more in common with humans than with plants. They have their own immune system and can produce vitamin D in their cells when exposed to the sun. Mushrooms are also clever. They can create an air flow around themserves which helps to spread their spores for future mushroom growth.

According to an ancient Greek myth, Perseus, while returning from a journey, drank river water by using the hat part of a mushroom. Later he founded a colony at that same spot and called it Mycenae, which is from the Greek word for mushroom (mykēs).

Traditional Chinese medicine uses mushrooms for their medicinal properties. They contain proteins, vitamins, minerals and antioxidants. These can have various health benefits.

POTATOES

Potato roots trace back to Peru where the Incas were the first to grow the crop 1,800 years ago. The Inca people once ruled a vast empire in the Indi mountains of South America. Their capital was Cuzco in what is now Peru. The Inca empire included around twelve million people at its peak in the early 1500s. Apart from potatoes, they grew other crops including corn, squash, tomatoes, peanuts and cotton. They also raised pigs, ducks, dogs and llamas.

Potatoes were introduced in Europe by Spain in 1536. Spanish tradition claims that Gonzalo Jiménez de Quesada was the first to introduce the potato in Europe, and that is probably why the word potato in Spanish is "patata".

It is said that the most famous potato dish, the French fry, was discovered by American soldiers in Belgium during the First World War. The dominant language of southern Belgium is French, and that is how this food received the name "French" fries. The French fry was allegedly served in the United States for the first time by Thomas Jefferson at a presidential dinner.

Today the world's largest potato producing country is China. Potatoes are among the most environmentally friendly vegetables. They are easy to grow and do not require any fertiliser or chemical additives to thrive. Potato plants are usually pollinated by insects such as bumblebees.

Despite their robust appearance, they are made up of 80% water and only 20% of solid. Even though they have a high content of water, potatoes are rich in compounds like flavonoids, carotenoids and phenolic acids. These compounds act as antioxidants in the body by neutralising potentially harmful molecules known as free radicals. When free radicals accumulate, they can increase the risk of chronic diseases like heart failure, diabetes and cancer.

ORANGES

Oranges and all citrus fruits originated in the southeast Himalayan foothills, in a region which includes eastern India, northern Myanmar and western China. A fossil specimen from Yunnan, China, provides evidence of the existence of citrus dating back to approximately eight million years ago.

The word "orange" first appeared in the English language in the twelfth century. It is thought to have originated via the old French word "orange". It is unclear if the name derived directly from Persian or Arabic, or whether it was imported from the Italian word "arancio" which means "orange tree".

An orange is a cross between a grapefruit and a mandarin. Its genes are about 25% grapefruit and about 75% mandarin. It probably dates back to 314 BC. Mention of it is found in Chinese literature dated to that period.

As of 1987, orange trees have been found to be the most cultivated fruit trees in the world. Brazil leads with 24% of the total world production, followed by China and India.

Orange juice tastes bad after brushing your teeth because toothpaste blocks your sweet taste receptors that are stimulated when tasting sweet fruits, including oranges. Oranges are very good for our health. They are a rich source of vitamin C, vitamin B, and minerals such as calcium, potassium, phosphorus and magnesium.

PUMPKINS

Indigenous North Americans have grown pumpkins for thousands of years, even before the cultivation of beans and corn. Pumpkins are actually a fruit and are members of the gourd family which includes cucumbers, honeydew melons, cantaloupe, watermelons and zucchini. The word pumpkin comes from the Greek word "pepon" which means a large melon.

Pumpkins are a nutrient-dense and naturally low-calorie food. They offer plenty of health benefits because they contain a high source of the antioxidant beta-carotene.

Every pumpkin produces about 500 seeds. Its bright orange colour and its green stems signal the transition from the hot summer season to the cooler, crisper air of autumn. It is also famously known as the mascot of the scariest and creepiest holiday of all, Halloween!

BROCCOLI

Broccoli have been around for more than 2000 years. They were mainly grown in Italy from the period of the Roman Empire until the sixteenth century when a royal marriage brought the vegetable to France.

The word "broccoli" comes from the Italian plural of "broccolo" which means "the flowering crest of a cabbage" and is the diminutive form of "brocco", meaning "small nail" or "sprout".

The health benefits of broccoli include their ability to prevent cancer, improve digestion, lower cholesterol levels, detoxify the body, and maximise vitamin and mineral intake. Broccoli also prevent allergic reactions, boost the immune system, protect the skin, prevent birth defects, lower blood pressure, eliminate inflammation, and improve eyesight.

APPLES

Archaeologists have found evidence that people have been eating apples since 6,500 BC. Apples originate from Kazakhstan, in Asia, east of the Caspian Sea. The name of the former capital of Kazakhstan, Almaty, is often translated as "full of apples". By 1500 BC, apple seeds had been carried throughout Europe. Later, Greeks and Romans cultivated apples and, during the early centuries of the Christian era, carried apple seeds and trees to the British Isles. Many varieties of apples thrived in England.

Apples are less dense than water. Therefore. they float in water because 25% of their volume is actually air. The top producing countries in the world are China, the United States, Turkey, Poland, and Italy. Most apples in the world are still picked by hand and, by volume, we eat more apples than any other fruit. They are a true symbol of autumn.

Apples are low in sodium, fat, and cholesterol, and are also a good source of vitamin C and fibre. Research shows that the antioxidants in apples can slow the growth of cancer cells, protecting the pancreas and lowering the chance of diabetes.

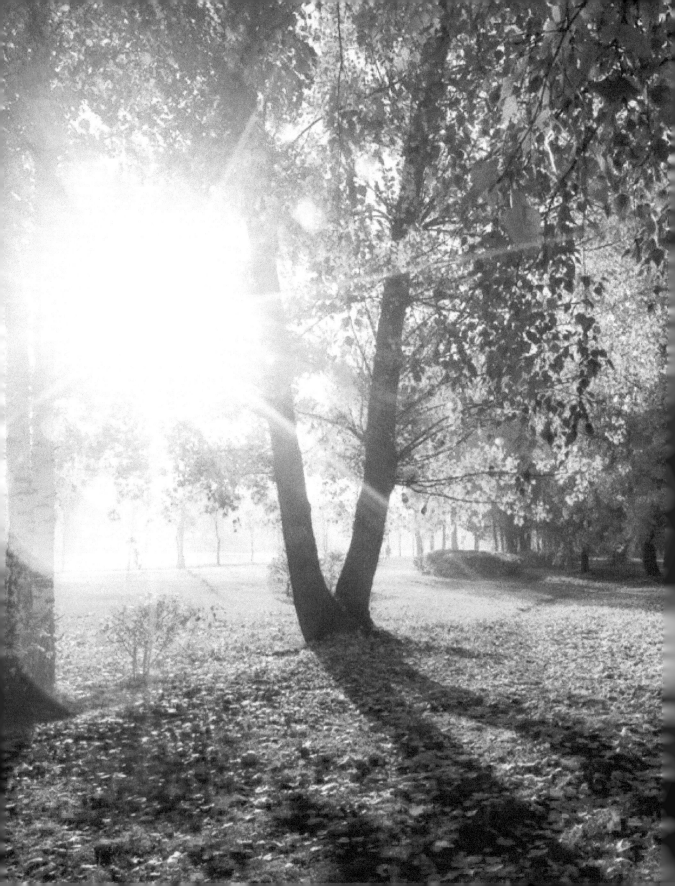

AUTUMN RECIPES

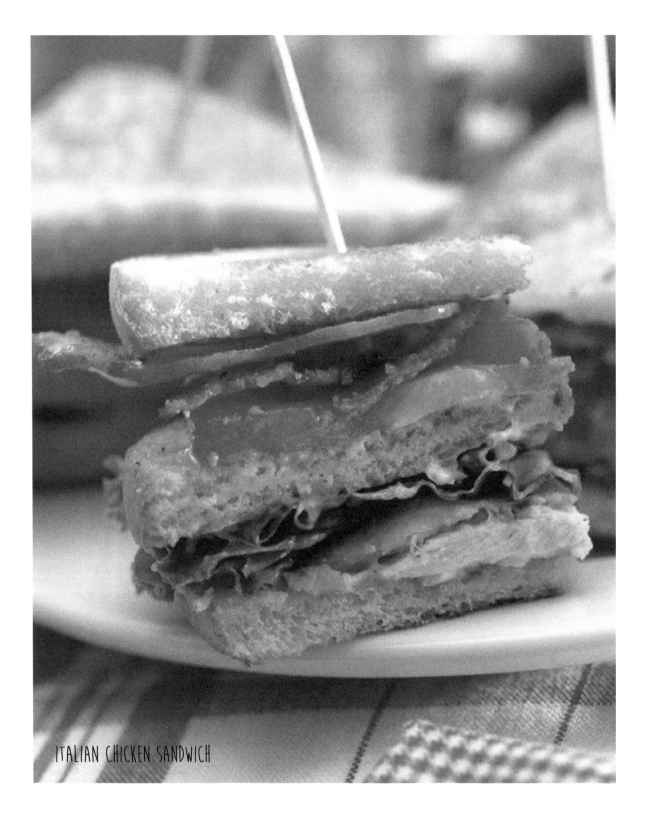

ITALIAN CHICKEN SANDWICH

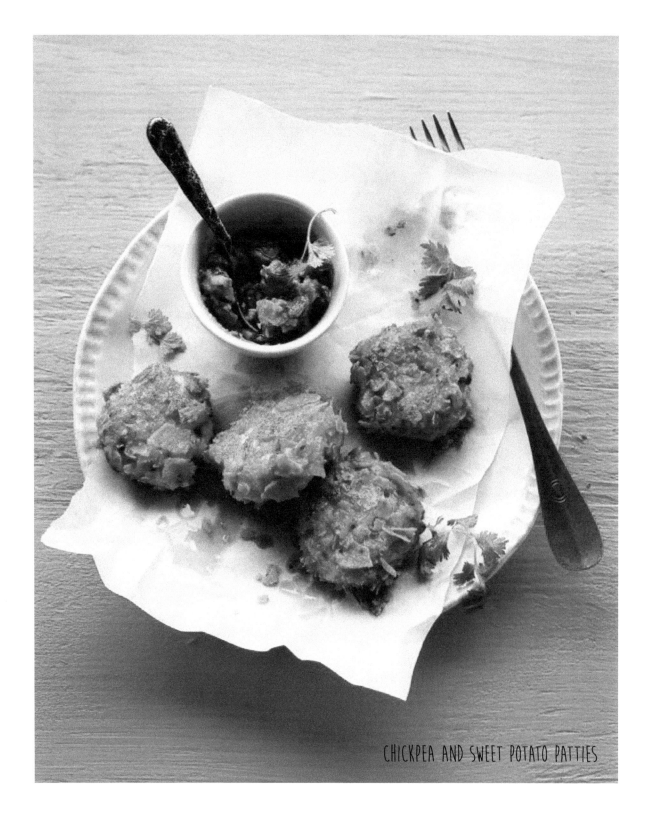

CHICKPEA AND SWEET POTATO PATTIES

ITALIAN CHICKEN SANDWICH
* * *
CHICKPEA AND SWEET POTATO PATTIES

SERVES TWO LUNCHBOXES

Italian chicken sandwich

- a handful of shredded iceberg lettuce
- 4 slices of Parma ham
- 4 slices of crusty, sour dough bread
- fresh, homemade or ready-made good-quality pesto
- chicken meat, cooked and shredded

Easy homemade pesto

- 2 tablespoons mixed pumpkin, sesame and sunflower seeds
- 1 cup packed fresh basil
- juice of 1 lemon
- ¼ cup olive oil to start (add if necessary)

Blend all the pesto ingredients until smooth. Add oil if necessary. Pour over the vegetable salad and stir until all the ingredients are evenly combined.

For the patties

- 1 sweet potato
- 100g chick peas
- 1 egg
- 2 teaspoons of grated parmesan
- a bunch of finely chopped coriander
- olive oil
- all-purpose flour

Fruit compartment

- 2 cups banana chips
- 2 cups blueberries
- 2 cups coconut chips

Sandwich assembly

Spread a small amount of pesto on the bread. Place the Parma ham on the first slice of bread. Arrange the lettuce and top with shredded chicken. Cover with the second slice of bread, press firmly to keep the ingredients together while slicing. Portion and place in a separate compartment of the lunchbox.

Chickpea and sweet potato patties

In a large mixing bowl using a potato masher, crush the chickpeas and a boiled sweet potato. Add parmesan, egg and finely chopped coriander. Mix well until you achieve a firm paste consistency.

Roll paste, using your hands, into small balls, and dip in flour. Flatten the balls to create a pattie and set aside. Drizzle a little olive oil in a pan and set on medium heat. Lower the patties in the hot oil without overcrowding. Repeat with the remaining mixture in batches to avoid reducing the temperature of the oil. Fry the patties for a couple of minutes on each side or until they turn golden brown, then remove them from the pan using a spoon, and transfer them onto a paper lined tray to drain.

Fruit compartment

Place a handful of blueberries in a lunchbox next to the banana chips and the coconut chips in three separate rows or mixed together as a fruit salad. You can have fun with fruit compartments, adding all kinds of dried fruits including pineapples, mangoes, raisins and cranberries. You may also add different kinds of berries or any seasonal fruit.

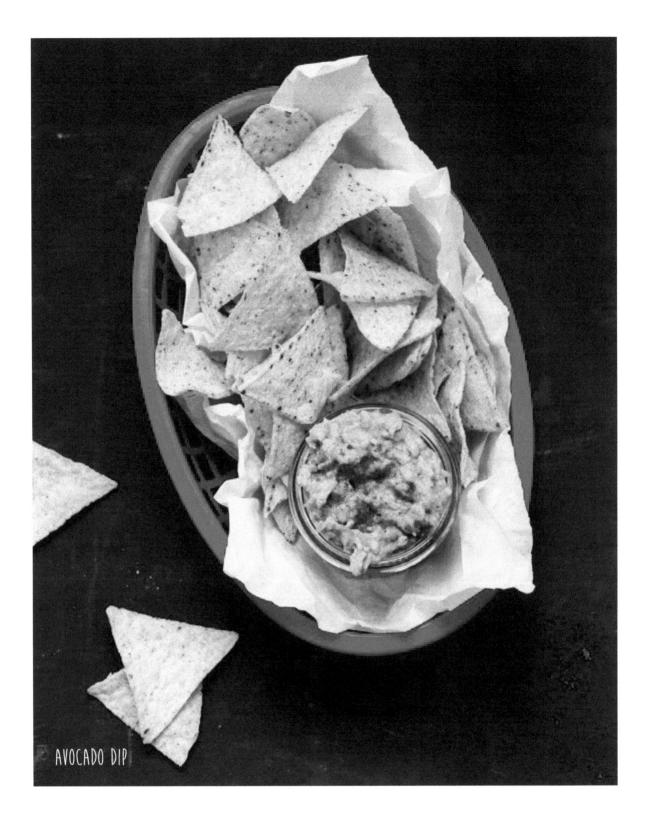

AVOCADO DIP

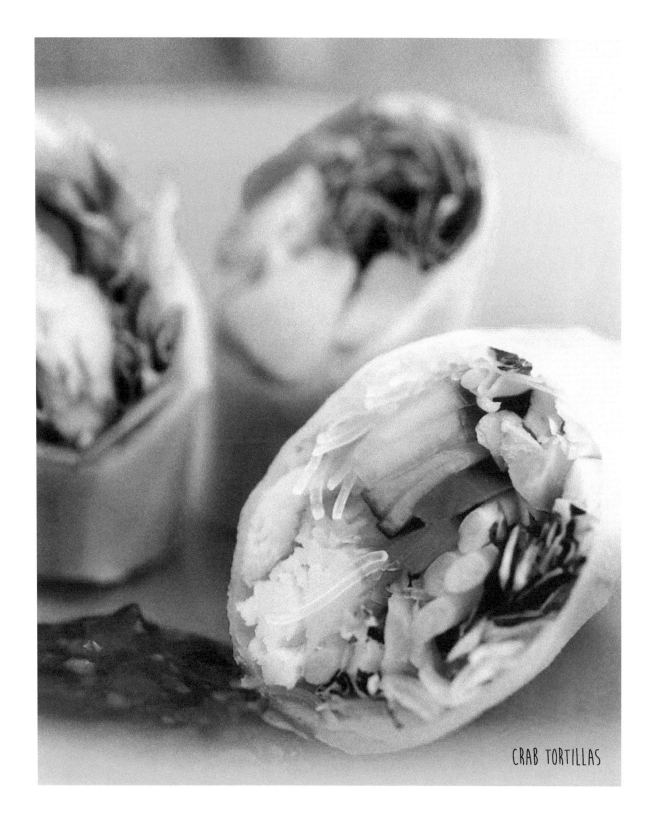

CRAB TORTILLAS

2
MEXICAN FIESTA
* * *
CRAB TORTILLAS AND AVOCADO DIP

SERVES TWO LUNCHBOXES

Crab tortillas

- *2 soft corn tortillas*
- *lettuce leaves*
- *2 cups, shredded carrots*
- *8 crab sticks or 50g leftover cooked fish*
- *cheese spread like Philadelphia*
- *bunch of coriander, finely chopped*

Salsa mix

- *1 cup frozen sweet corn, defrosted*
- *1 cup cherry tomatoes*
- *2 carrots, peeled and cut in sticks*

Avocado dip

- *1 avocado*
- *juice of half a lime*
- *salt and pepper*
- *finely chopped parsley*
- *a handful of corn chips for each lunchbox*

Tortilla assembly

Tortillas are easier to handle when they are heated for a couple of minutes in a hot oven. Spread some Philadelphia cheese, place some lettuce and add the shredded carrots. Arrange the crab sticks in the middle and sprinkle some finely chopped coriander. Fold the top and bottom ends to secure the ingredients. Roll tightly and portion.

Salsa mix

Place a handful of sweet corn, a handful of cherry tomatoes and carrot sticks in a separate compartment of the lunchbox next to the avocado dip.

Avocado dip

Cut the avocado in halves. Remove the stones and discard. Scoop out the flesh and tip in a fruit processor with the lime juice and parsley. Season well with salt and pepper and blend until smooth. Serve alongside some organic corn chips.

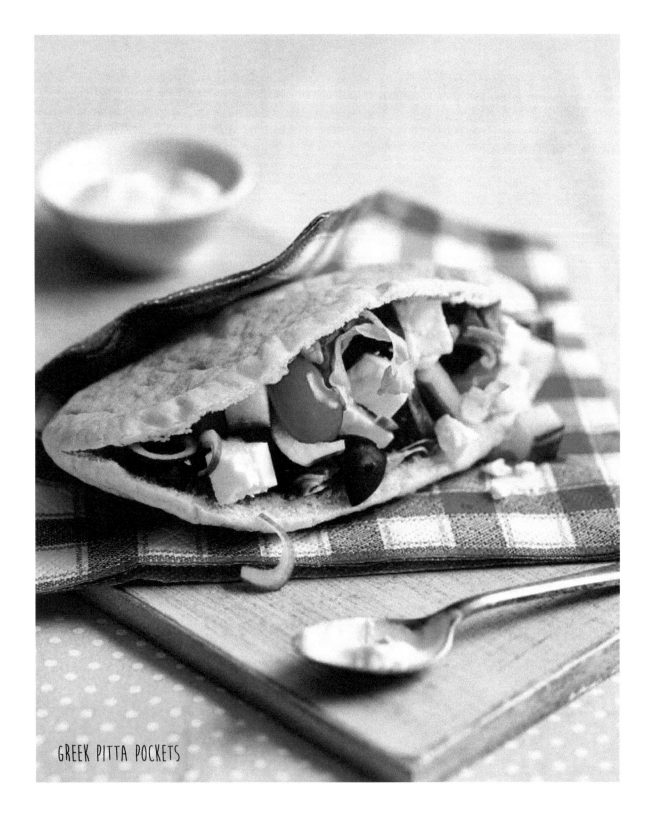

GREEK PITTA POCKETS

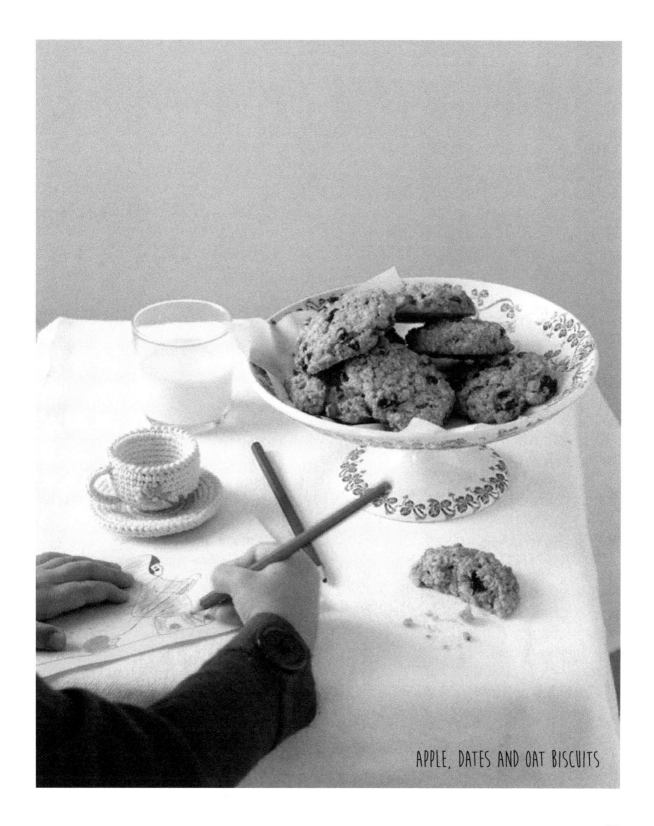

APPLE, DATES AND OAT BISCUITS

39

3

GREEK PITTA POCKETS AND VEGETABLES STICKS
✳ ✳ ✳
APPLE, DATES AND OAT BISCUITS

SERVES TWO LUNCHBOXES

Pitta pockets

- *6 mini party-size pitta pockets*
- *a handful of shredded lettuce*
- *2 tomatoes*
- *½ cucumber*
- *60g lactose-free feta cheese*
- *olive oil*
- *dried oregano*
- *carrot, coloured peppers and cucumber sticks (enough for two lunchboxes)*

Spiced hummus

- *200g chickpeas, cooked as per packet instructions*
- *fresh turmeric, finely grated*
- *1 clove garlic*
- *1 teaspoon cumin seeds, toasted and crushed*
- *juice and zest of 1 lemon*
- *4 teaspoons tahini*
- *olive oil*

Apple and dates

- *2 apples, cut in quarters*
- *lemon juice*
- *unpitted dates*

Oat biscuits

- *75g wholemeal flour*
- *1 teaspoon baking powder*
- *75g porridge oats*
- *50g brown sugar*
- *75g butter*
- *½ tablespoon maple syrup*
- *½ tablespoon golden syrup*
- *2 tablespoons vanilla-flavoured plant-based milk*

Oat biscuits

Heat the oven to 180°C. Line a baking tray with baking paper. Sift the flour into a bowl mixing baking powder, porridge oats, and sugar. Melt the butter syrup and the milk in a small saucepan or in the microwave and stir. Add the dry ingredients and mix until the liquid covers all the oat mixture and until the ingredients are evenly combined. Spoon onto a baking tray and shape into rounds leaving space between each biscuit as they will spread while cooking. Bake for 10 to 15 minutes or until they turn golden brown. Leave to cool for 5 minutes before removing from tray.

Apple and dates

Cut the apple in quarters. Keep the peel on but remove all the seeds. Squeeze some lemon juice on the apples so that they do not brown. Place in one of the lunchbox compartments together with some unpitted dates.

Pitta assembly

Create a pocket in the pitta bread by cutting a small opening on the top edge. Make a Greek salad mixture by adding the lettuce, tomato slices, cucumber slices, feta cubes, oregano and olive oil. Stir well and place inside the pitta pocket.

Vegetable sticks

Chop the carrot, cucumber or celery and coloured peppers in sticks. This may be done the night before and stored in an airtight container immersed in water.

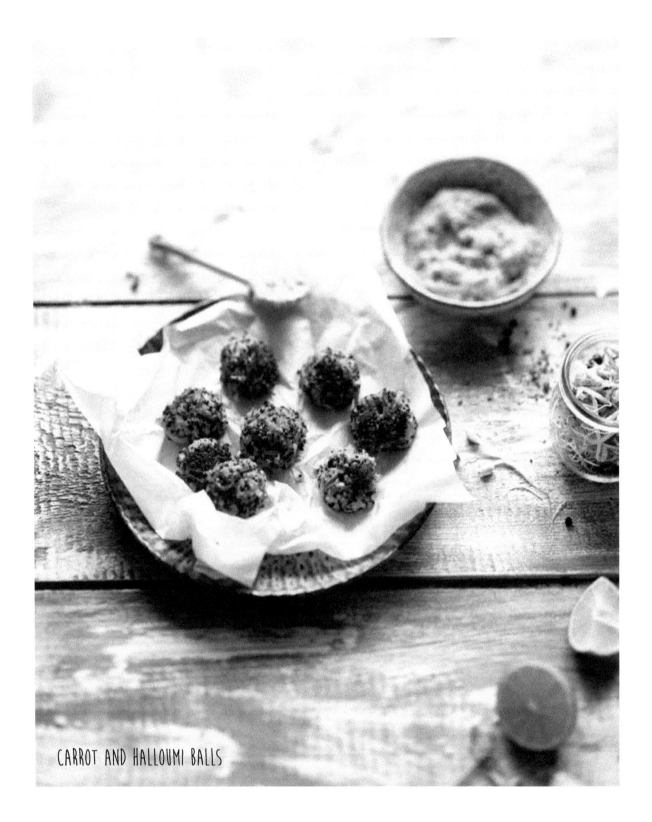

CARROT AND HALLOUMI BALLS

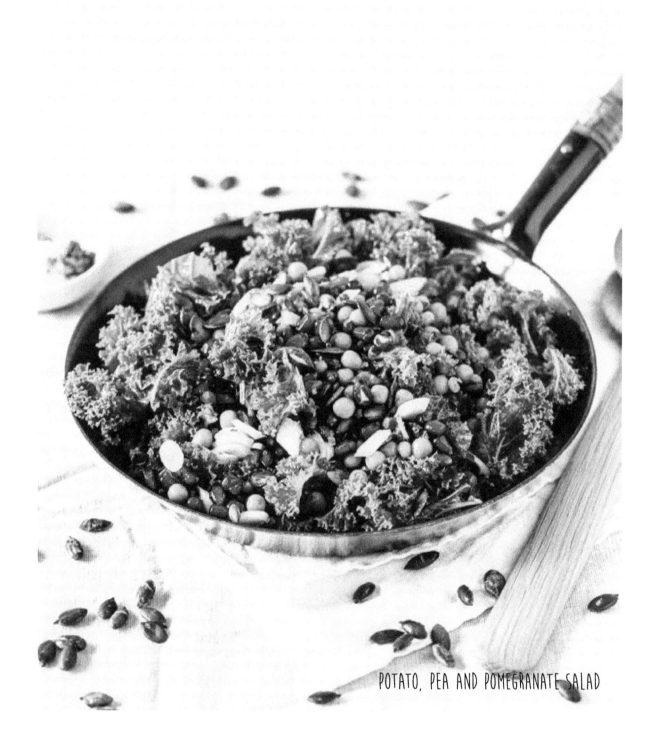

POTATO, PEA AND POMEGRANATE SALAD

43

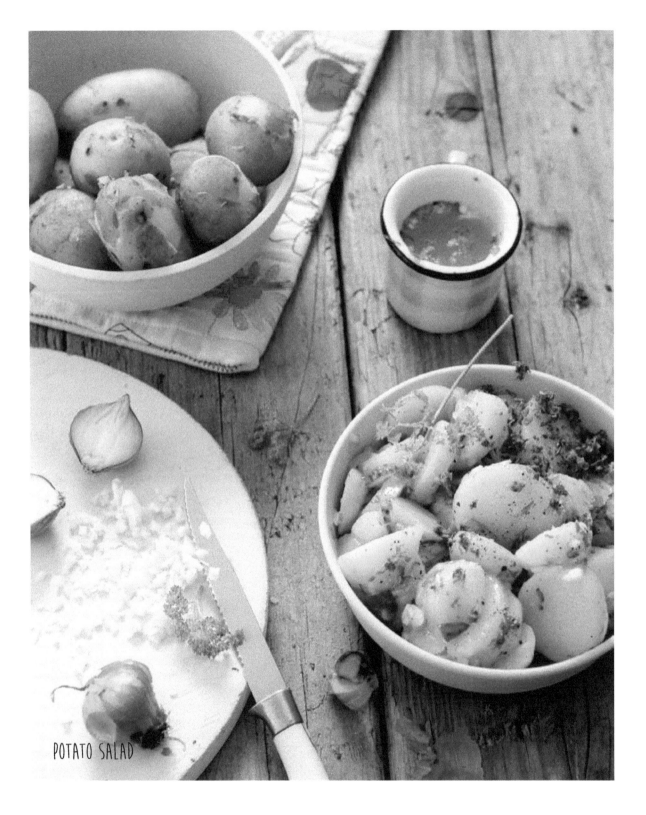

POTATO SALAD

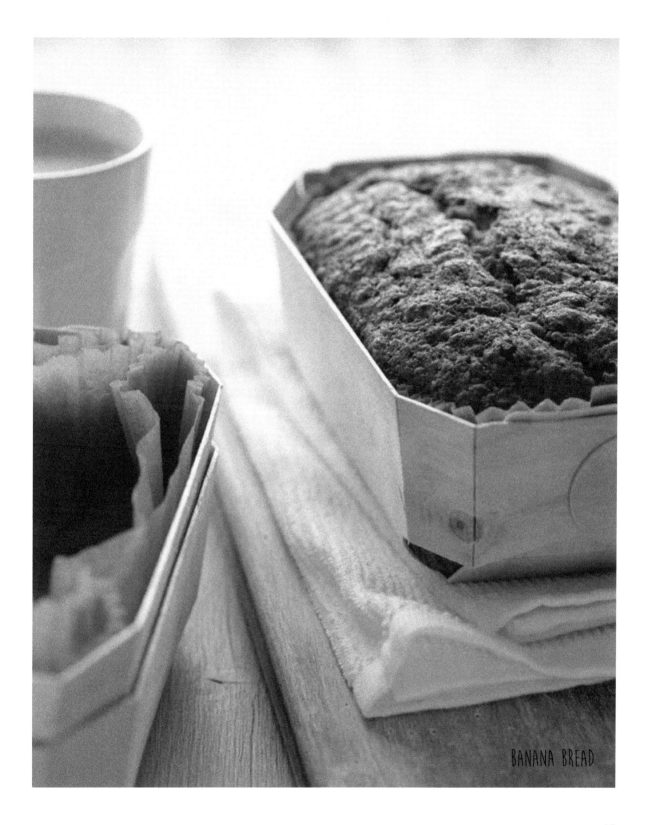

BANANA BREAD

4

CARROT AND HALLOUMI BALLS
***
POTATO, PEA AND POMEGRANATE SALAD
***
ORANGE, CREAMY DESSERT WITH BANANA BREAD

SERVES TWO LUNCHBOXES

Carrot, halloumi balls

- *1 carrot, peeled and grated coarsely*
- *125g halloumi cheese, grated coarsely*
- *1 egg*
- *2 tablespoons plain flour*
- *cumin seeds, paprika, salt and pepper*
- *olive oil*

Potato salad

- *2 potatoes, boiled and diced*
- *olive oil*
- *finely chopped parsley*
- *juice of ½ lemon, freshly squeezed*
- *salt and pepper*

Peas and pomegranate

- *a handful of frozen peas for each lunchbox*
- *a handful of pomegranate seeds for each lunchbox*

Fruit compartment

- *2 oranges*
- *2 organic yoghurts of choice*

Banana bread

- *60g butter, melted*
- *⅔ cup castor sugar*
- *2 bananas*
- *1 egg*
- *1½ cup of self-raising flour*
- *½ cup vanilla-flavoured plant-based milk (if using regular milk, add 1 teaspoon of vanilla essence)*

Carrot halloumi balls

Line a plate with cooking paper and put aside. Place the grated carrots and halloumi along with the remaining ingredients into a mixing bowl. Season well with salt, pepper and the rest of the spices, and work mixture with your hands to combine evenly.

Meanwhile, heat some olive oil in a pan. Using your hands, roll spoonfuls of mixture into balls. Carefully lower the balls into the hot pan and cook in batches for 3 to 4 minutes until golden brown. When cooked, place on paper lined plate to drain excess oil.

Potato salad

Place the diced boiled potato in a bowl. Squeeze the lemon and add a little olive oil and the finely chopped parsley. Season well with salt and pepper, and mix well very gently not to break the potatoes.

Peas and pomegranate

In a separate lunchbox compartment, place the boiled peas, and top with a handful of pomegranate. Season well with salt and pepper.

Banana bread

Preheat the oven to 175°C. Grease a loaf pan, and line with parchment paper. Combine sugar and flour. In a separate bowl, whisk the egg and the mashed banana, and stir until combined well. Add the melted butter, milk and dry ingredients. Mix until evenly combined. Pour the batter into the loaf pan and bake in the hot oven for about 20-30 minutes until golden brown and a skewer inserted in the middle comes out clean.

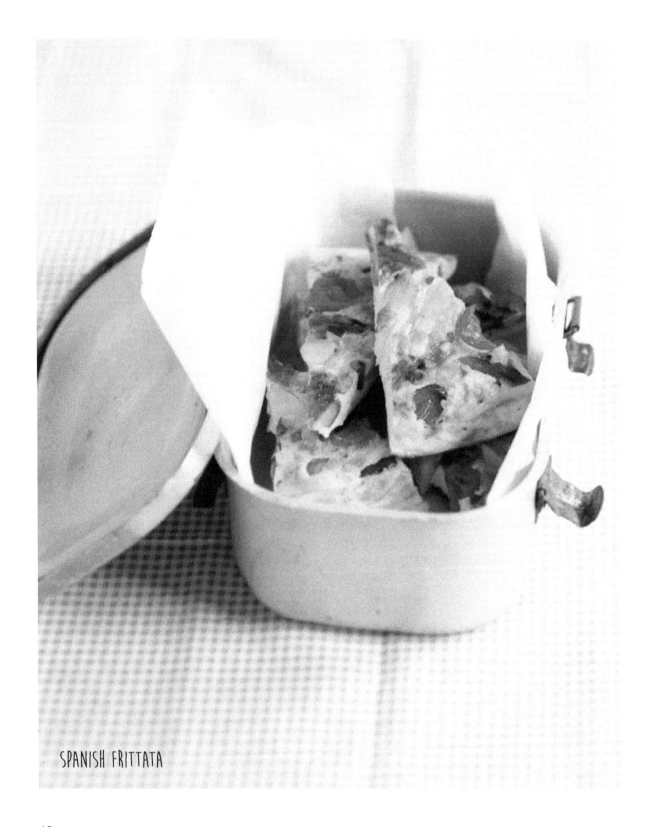

SPANISH FRITTATA

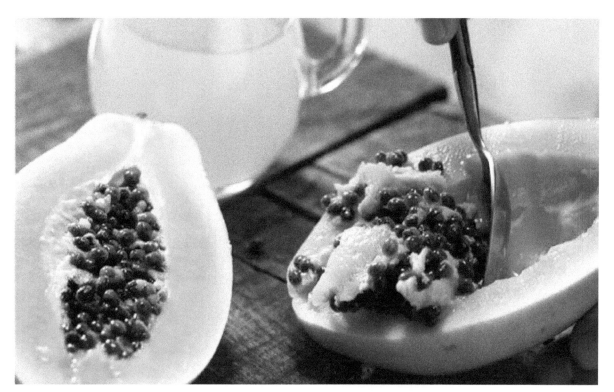

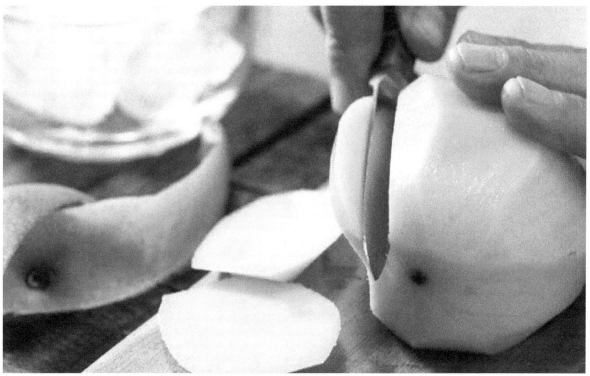

5

SPANISH FRITTATA
* * *
EDAMAME AND RICE CRACKERS
* * *
VIETNAMESE STIR-FRY NOODLES
* * *
MANGO AND PAPAYA

SERVES TWO LUNCHBOXES

Spanish frittata

- *olive oil*
- *½ of a spring onion*
- *½ cup cooked potatoes, cut into cubes*
- *½ cup red peppers, cut in small cubes*
- *pinch of paprika*
- *bunch of finely-chopped parsley*
- *2 eggs, beaten*
- *½ cup shredded hard cheese*
- *2 slices chorizo, finely chopped in small cubes (optional)*

Condiments

- *frozen edamame beans boiled for a few minutes, drained and salted*
- *rice crackers or rice cakes or prawn crackers*

Vietnamese stir-fry noodles

- *100g egg noodles*
- *a few broccoli florets*
- *2 tablespoons fish sauce*
- *1 tablespoon rice vinegar*
- *1 teaspoon brown sugar*
- *1 tablespoon oyster sauce*
- *1 tablespoon water*
- *1 tablespoon vegetable oil*
- *finely-chopped spring onion*
- *½ red pepper, finely chopped*
- *1 carrot, thinly sliced*
- *50g mushrooms*
- *few snap peas or mangetout*
- *a bunch of coriander leaves*

Mango and papaya

- *1 mango, peeled and cut in chunks*
- *1 papaya, peeled, deseeded and cut in chunks*

Cut the fruit in similar size and place neatly in a separate compartment of the lunchbox. Squeeze some fresh lime juice.

Spanish frittata

Heat some olive oil in a skillet, add the spring onions, potatoes and peppers and fry until tender and golden. Add the chorizo, if using, paprika and parsley and stir until combined. Add the eggs and season with salt and pepper. Let the mixture cook until the eggs are set, stirring occasionally to prevent them from sticking to the pan. Sprinkle the cheese over the frittata. Then place the pan under a preheated grill until the cheese is melted. Remove from under the grill and set aside to cool. Once the frittata cools enough to handle, cut into quarters or bite-size cubes and place in a separate lunchbox compartment lined with baking paper.

Vietnamese stir-fry noodles

In a bowl mix together the fish sauce, the vinegar, the sugar, the oyster sauce and the water. Before starting the stir-fry, make sure that all the ingredients are prepared as there will be no time to do so during the cooking process. Heat some vegetable oil in a wok and toss all the ingredients on high heat for a few minutes until the vegetables are tender, and set aside. Meanwhile, boil some water, drop in the broccoli and noodles and cook for just over 3 minutes. Remove from the boiling water and add to the stir-fry vegetables. Add the previously mixed sauces and combine well, making sure that the vegetables are well coated with the sauce. Garnish with coriander and let it set for the flavours to be absorbed by the noodles.

When placing in a separate compartment in the lunchbox, make sure you drain the noodles of any liquid.

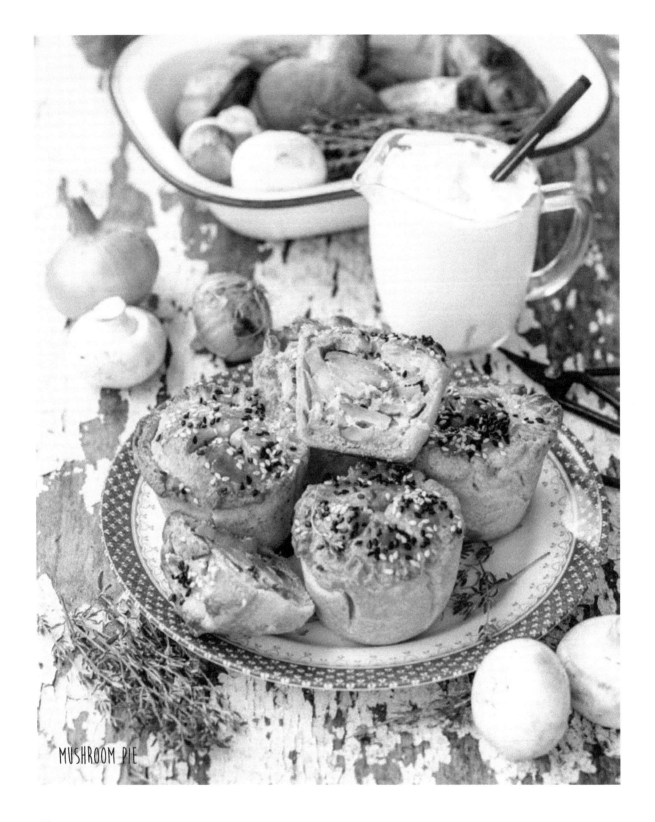

MUSHROOM PIE

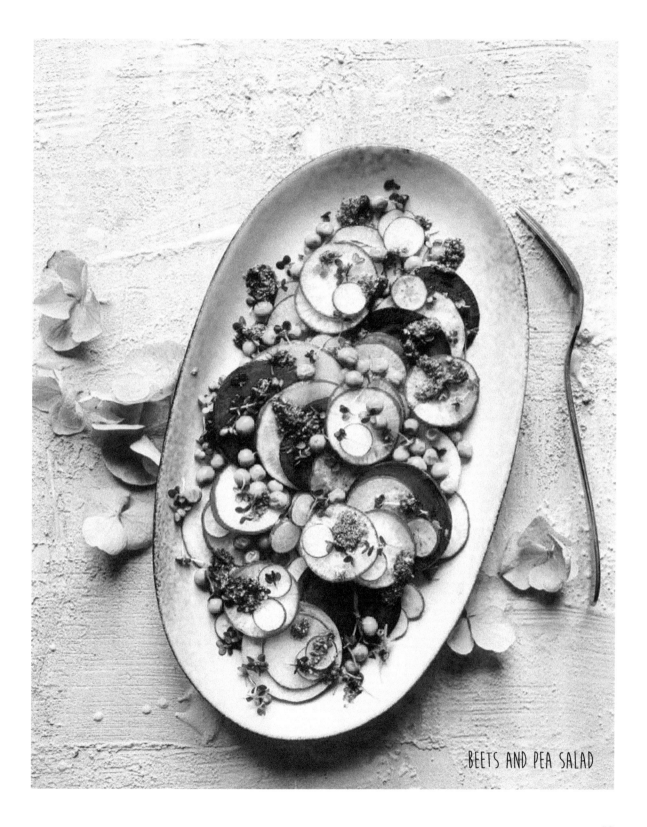

BEETS AND PEA SALAD

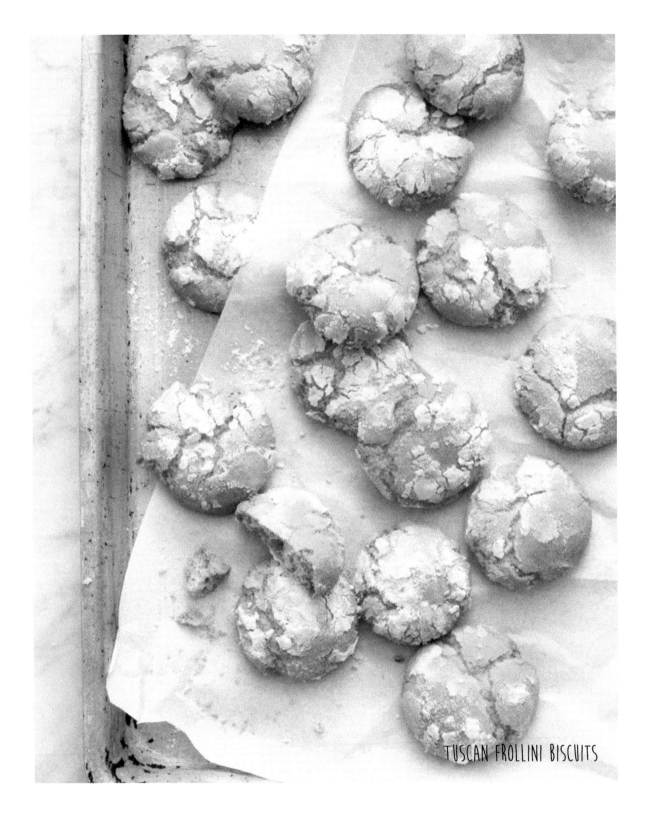

TUSCAN FROLLINI BISCUITS

6

MUSHROOM PIE
✳ ✳ ✳
BEETS AND PEA SALAD
✳ ✳ ✳
TUSCAN FROLLINI BISCUITS WITH BLACKBERRY RIPPLES

—————————— • ——————————

SERVES TWO LUNCHBOXES

Mushroom pie

- *½ an onion*
- *½ a leek*
- *350g mushrooms*
- *thyme*
- *rosemary*
- *olive oil*
- *2 pastry sheets, ready rolled*
- *puff pastry or short crust*
- *béchamel of choice or make your own*
- *1 tablespoon olive oil*
- *2 tablespoons plain flour*
- *225ml of skimmed milk, lactose free or plant-based milk*

Beets and pea salad

- *4 beetroots, fresh*
- *olive oil*
- *balsamic vinegar*
- *rosemary*
- *1 teaspoon brown sugar*
- *1 cup frozen peas*
- *12 green beans, cleaned from stem at the edges*
- *50g feta cheese*

Tuscan frollini biscuits

These biscuits are an old Tuscan recipe passed on through generations since the time of the famous poet Dante Alighieri. These biscuits are tender and indulgent. They are a perfect treat to break the day.

Makes 24 biscuits. (Uncooked dough freezes well. If frozen in portions, you can bake as many biscuits as required.)

- *220g flour 00*
- *1 egg*
- *125g butter*
- *70g castor sugar*
- *1 tablespoon finely grated lemon zest*

Blackberry ripple

- *100g blackberries, fresh or frozen*
- *25g icing sugar*
- *80g Greek yoghurt*

Mushroom pies

Prepare the vegetables by finely chopping the onion. Trim and thinly slice the leek, quarter the mushrooms, and remove the leaves from the herbs by running your fingers from the top to the base of the stem. The leaves should easily come away. Chop them finely.

Put the frying pan over medium heat and add the olive oil. Cook the onion, the leek, the mushrooms and the herbs for a few minutes, stirring occasionally. Season and increase the heat until the mushrooms are soft and all the liquid has evaporated. Remove from the heat and set aside.

To make the best béchamel, put the saucepan over medium heat and add the oil and the flour, and stir vigorously for two or three minutes. Gradually add the milk, whisking constantly until smooth.

Bring to the boil, then simmer for two minutes until thick. Merge half the mushroom mixture with a blender until smooth. Then add all the rest of the mushrooms to the pan with the smoothened mushroom blend and béchamel and stir well until everything is well combined. Season if necessary. If using a ready-made béchamel, heat before mixing with the mushrooms.

Unroll the pastry sheets and cut out six 10 cm circles. Lightly press into the muffin holes so that there is some excess pastry out of the mould. Divide the mushroom filling between the muffin holes, and cut out six circles of unrolled pastry. Top the pies with the circle, pressing the pastry tightly to seal, and secure the edges with a fork. Brush with olive oil or a beaten egg and bake for 25 to 30 minutes or until golden and crispy. Let the pies cool completely before placing them in a separate compartment in the lunchbox.

Beets and pea salad

Boil the frozen peas and the cleaned green beans until cooked but still firm. Drain and set aside. Preheat the oven to 200°C. Peel the beetroots and cut into wedges. Put in a bowl with the rosemary, oil, vinegar and sugar, and season well. Stir until the beetroots are well coated.

Tip the coated beetroots in a roasting tin and roast in the oven for 30-40 minutes until tender.

When the beetroots have completely cooled, cut them in smaller cubes. In a bowl, mix the beetroots with the cooked green beans and the peas, and combine well. Place in a compartment in the lunchbox and top with the crushed feta cheese.

Tuscan frollini biscuits

Mix by hand, or by using an electric mixer, the flour, sugar, butter, egg and lemon zest until you obtain a smooth ball of dough. Cover the dough in a kitchen towel and leave to rest in the refrigerator for 30 minutes.

Meanwhile, line a baking dish with a non-stick baking sheet and preheat the oven to 200°C. Once the dough is ready to use, roll 24 balls using your hands, and place in the prepared baking dish leaving some space between them. Flatten gently with the back of a teaspoon and bake for 20 minutes until the biscuits are lightly golden. Take out of the oven and let the biscuits cool completely before removing them from the baking dish.

Blackberry ripple

Put aside four whole blackberries. Place the remaining berries in a liquidiser with the icing sugar. Blend until well combined but not too watery. Mix half of the liquidised berries with the Greek yoghurt.

Place the remaining berry mixture at the bottom of a compartment in the lunchbox. Top with the Greek yoghurt mixture to create separate layers. Decorate on top with two whole blackberries.

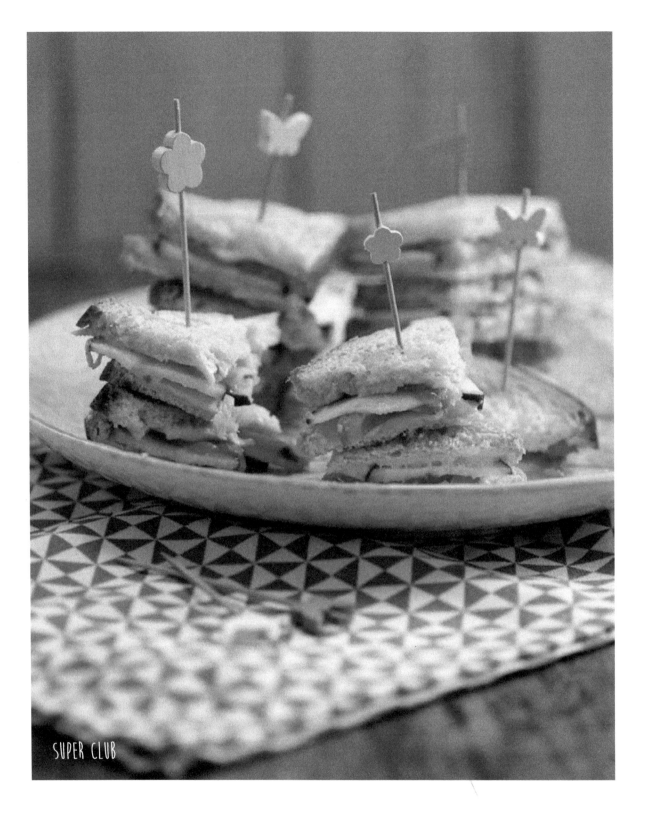

SUPER CLUB

58

7
SUPER CLUB
✳ ✳ ✳
CHEESE AND OAT CAKE
✳ ✳ ✳
BANANA AND CITRUS SALAD

SERVES TWO LUNCHBOXES

Super club

- *¼ cup cream cheese*
- *1 teaspoon of honey mustard*
- *4 slices wholegrain bread*
- *2 slices deli sliced roasted ham*
- *2 slices deli sliced turkey*
- *40g hard cheese, thinly sliced*
- *1 tomato, thinly sliced*
- *1 avocado, mashed*

Condiments

- *a few cubes of hard cheese (comte, parmigiano reggiano, grana padano and/or manchego)*

Place the cheese in a separate compartment of the lunchbox together with some crackers or oatcakes.

Banana and citrus salad

- *1 banana*
- *1 orange*
- *1 grapefruit*
- *mint, finely chopped*
- *juice of half a lemon*
- *drizzle of clear honey*

Super club

Combine the cream cheese and mustard in a small bowl and spread the mixture over the first slice of bread. Add the ham and the turkey. Arrange the tomato over the filling and top with the cheese. Spread the mashed avocado over the second slice of bread and cover the rest of the ingredients, gently pressing the bread to keep all the ingredients secure while slicing.

Banana and citrus salad

Peel and chop the banana in thin slices. Peel and deseed the orange and the grapefruit and segment in supremes. Tip the fruit in a bowl with finely chopped mint, lemon juice and a drizzle of clear honey. Stir well to combine all the flavours until all the flavours coat the fruit.

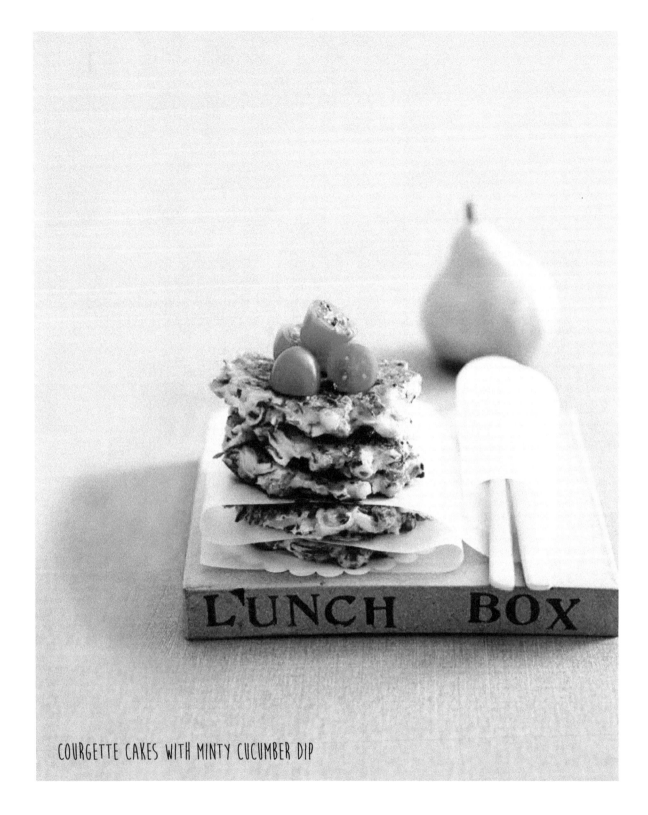

COURGETTE CAKES WITH MINTY CUCUMBER DIP

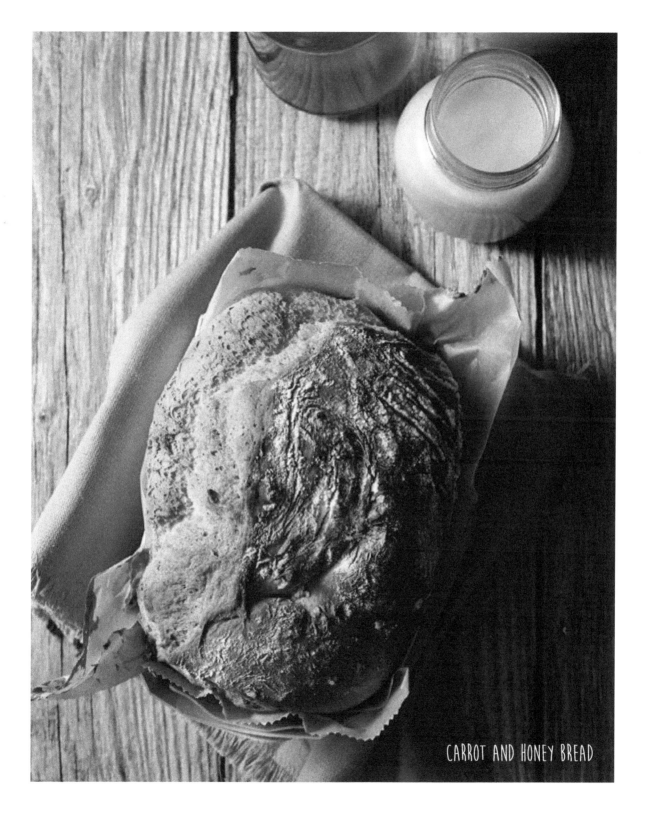

CARROT AND HONEY BREAD

8

COURGETTE CAKES WITH MINTY CUCUMBER DIP
***
VEGETABLE STICKS, APPLES AND DATES
***
CARROT AND HONEY BREAD

SERVES TWO LUNCHBOXES

Courgette cakes with minty cucumber dip

- *350g grated courgettes*
- *1 potato, boiled and roughly mashed*
- *100g feta cheese*
- *a handful of finely-chopped spring onion*
- *a bunch of mint and dill, finely chopped*
- *1 tablespoon black sesame seeds*
- *100g panko breadcrumbs*
- *2 eggs, beaten*
- *sunflower oil*
- *150g good-quality tzatziki*

Condiments

- *deseeded and sliced coloured peppers*
- *peeled and sliced carrot sticks*
- *½ cucumber, deseeded and chopped in sticks*
- *2 apples*
- *4 dates*

Chop up all the vegetables and place in a separate compartment close to tzatziki dip. In a separate compartment, place the quartered apple and top with the dates.

Carrot and honey bread

- *25g butter*
- *½ cup honey*
- *¼ cup light brown sugar*
- *2 cups all-purpose flour*
- *2 teaspoons baking powder*
- *1 teaspoon ground cinnamon*
- *1 cup muesli*
- *2 carrots, grated*
- *¾ cup chopped dates*
- *⅓ cup golden raisins*
- *1 egg*
- *½ cup milk*
- *3 tablespoons sunflower seeds*

Courgette cakes with minty cucumber dip

Place the grated courgettes into a sieve and sprinkle with a very generous pinch of salt and leave them to drain for about an hour. Place the courgettes in a tea towel and squeeze all the liquid out. Meanwhile, place the cooled potato mash in a mixing bowl with the remaining ingredients, apart from the oil, adding the grated courgettes at the end. Stir the ingredients until evenly combined. Using your hands, shape the mixture into small cakes and set aside in the refrigerator for 30 minutes.

To coat the cakes, roll first in the egg mixture and then in the breadcrumbs, frying them in batches in the sunflower oil for two to three minutes until golden brown.

For the tzatziki dip, simply stir some finely chopped mint in good-quality ready-made tzatziki and sprinkle with olive oil.

Carrot and honey bread

Preheat the oven at 180°C. Grease a loaf pan with a little oil and line the bottom with non-stick parchment paper. Put the butter, honey and sugar into a saucepan and heat gently stirring until the butter has melted and the sugar has dissolved. Remove from the heat and set aside to cool.

Put the flour, baking powder, cinnamon and muesli in a bowl and mix together. Add the grated carrots and golden raisins, and mix with the rest of the ingredients until evenly combined. Finally, pour the honey mixture, eggs and milk and combine until smooth.

Spoon the batter into the prepared pan, level the surface, and sprinkle with sunflower seeds. Bake in the preheated oven for about an hour until the top has cracked slightly and is golden brown. A skewer must come out clean when inserted in the centre of the bread.

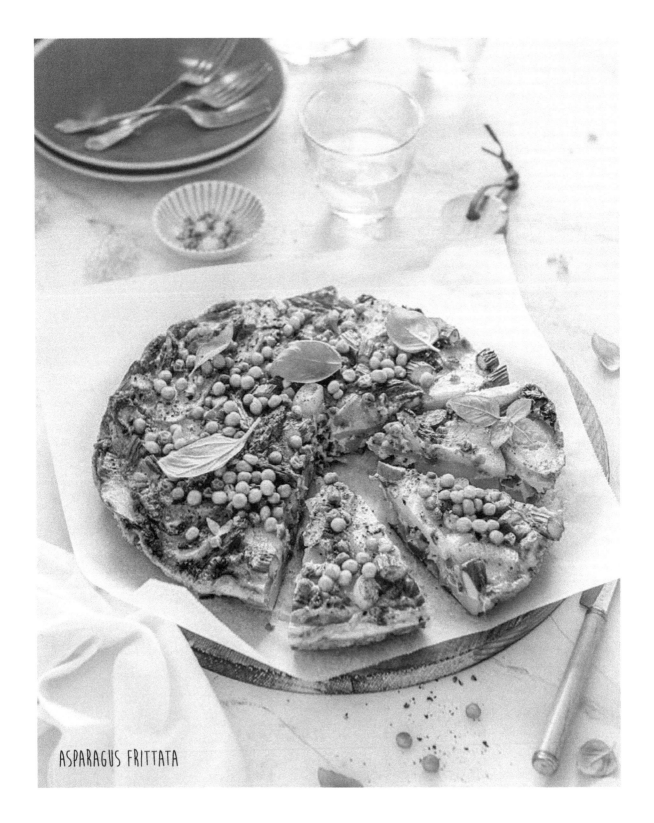

ASPARAGUS FRITTATA

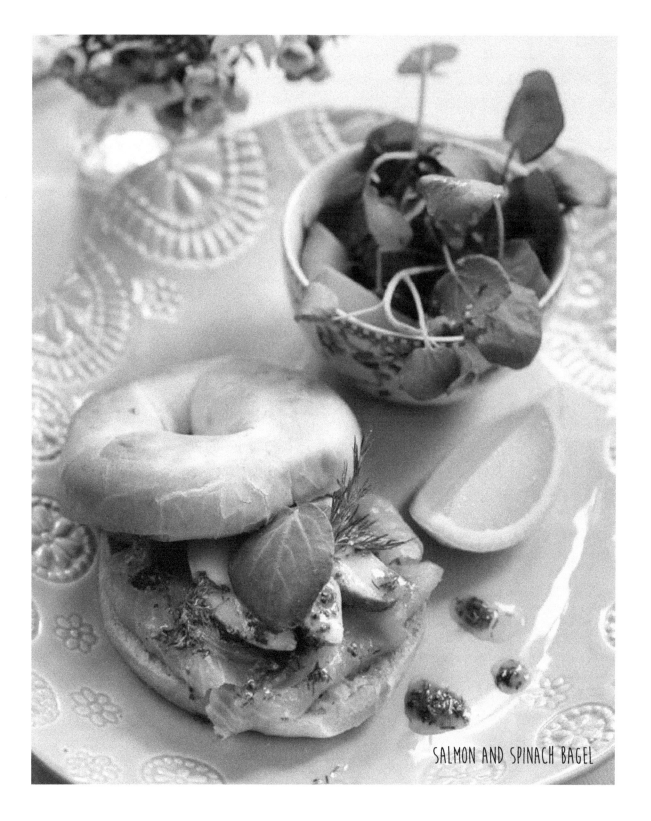

SALMON AND SPINACH BAGEL

9

ASPARAGUS FRITTATA
* * *
AVOCADO AND TOMATO SALAD
* * *
SALMON AND SPINACH BAGEL
* * *
KIWI, PEAR AND GRAPES

SERVES TWO LUNCHBOXES

Asparagus frittata

- *3 eggs*
- *5 asparagus stalks*
- *olive oil*

Avocado and tomato salad

- *1 avocado peeled, destoned and chopped in chunks*
- *1 tomato chopped in chunks*
- *bunch basil, finely chopped*
- *olive oil*
- *juice of half a lemon*

To make the salad, add all the ingredients in a bowl and stir to combine all the flavours. Season with salt and pepper, and place in a compartment of the lunchbox.

Kiwi, pear and grapes

- *2 crisp tart eating pears, cut in thin slices*
- *2 firm kiwis, cut in thin slices*
- *handful of green grapes, deseeded and halved*
- *¼ cup of lemon juice*

To make the salad, place the chopped fruit in a separate compartment of the lunchbox. Top with a drizzle of honey and lemon juice.

Salmon and spinach bagel

- *1 bagel per lunchbox*
- *4 smoked salmon slices*
- *1 tablespoon of chive-flavoured cream cheese*
- *a bunch of baby spinach leaves*

Asparagus frittata

Wash the asparagus, remove the base and finely chop the rest of the stalks. In a small bowl, beat the eggs with a fork and season with salt and pepper. Add the asparagus and stir until the asparagus are coated with the egg mixture.

Heat a pan with some olive oil and cook the omelette on medium heat until golden brown. Flip the omelette and repeat the process on the other side. It should take about 5 minutes on either side.

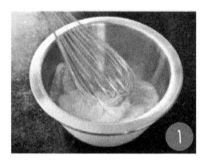 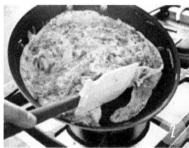 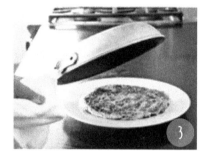

Salmon and spinach bagel

If your bagels are frozen, defrost and heat for a few minutes in a hot oven. Spread the chive-flavoured cream cheese and lay the smoked salmon and spinach over the bagel base. Place the second half of the bagel over the filling and press gently to fix the ingredients in place.

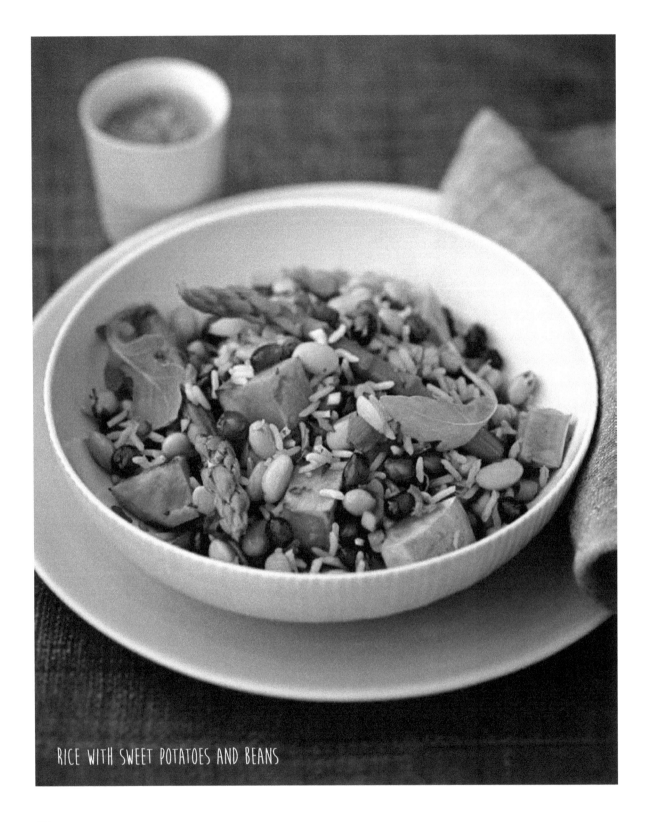

RICE WITH SWEET POTATOES AND BEANS

10

RICE WITH SWEET POTATOES AND BEANS
✳ ✳ ✳
FIBRE-PACKED FRUIT SALAD

SERVES TWO LUNCHBOXES

Rice with sweet potatoes and beans

- *2 sweet potatoes*
- *olive oil*
- *½ teaspoon mild chilli*
- *200g kidney beans*
- *200ml coconut milk*
- *100g long grain rice*
- *¼ teaspoon allspice*
- *bunch of coriander, finely chopped*
- *1 avocado, chopped in chunks*

Fibre-packed fruit salad

- *2 kiwis*
- *handful of dried banana slices for each lunchbox*
- *2 pots Greek yoghurt*
- *zest of half a lime*
- *a handful of coconut chips*
- *drizzle of honey*

Rice with sweet potatoes and beans

First cook the sweet potatoes. Peel them and cut them into two centimetre chunks. Spread them over a baking tray with a splash of olive oil. Sprinkle mild chilli and season with salt and pepper. Roast for 25 to 30 minutes, turning halfway. Meanwhile, make the rice and beans. Put the saucepan over medium heat, add the coconut milk to 100ml water and bring to a simmer. Wash the rice under cold water until it runs clear, and tip into the saucepan. Stir, reduce the heat to a gentle simmer, put the lid on, and cook until the liquid has been absorbed. This will take around 15 minutes. Take the pan off the heat and fold in the kidney beans.

Place the rice in one of the lunchbox compartments, add the roasted sweet potatoes on top, and garnish with the finely chopped coriander.

Fibre-packed fruit salad

Peel and slice the kiwis and place neatly in a row in a separate lunchbox compartment. In another compartment, tip a handful of banana chips. In a small mixing bowl, stir lime zest and honey with the Greek yoghurt. Place in an airtight container of the lunchbox and sprinkle some coconut chips on top.

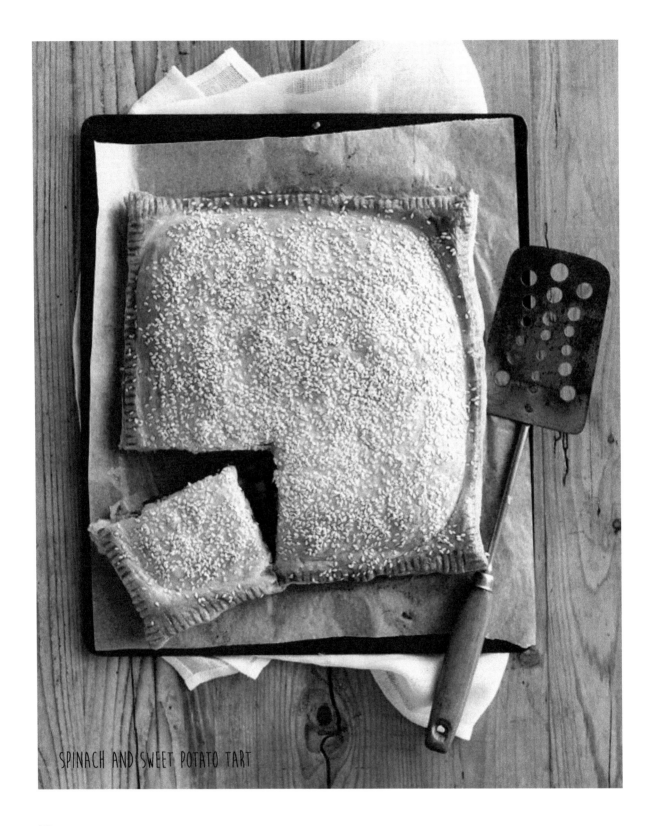

SPINACH AND SWEET POTATO TART

11

SPINACH AND SWEET POTATO TART
✻ ✻ ✻
EDAMAME AND APPLE
✻ ✻ ✻
BLUEBERRY MUFFINS

SERVES TWO LUNCHBOXES

Spinach and sweet potato tart

- *300g sweet potato, peeled and boiled*
- *150g spinach*
- *2 eggs, beaten*
- *1 cup ricotta*
- *½ cup grated parmesan*
- *2 sheets good-quality ready-made short crust pastry*

Condiments

- *Edamame, cooked as per packet instructions*
- *2 apples cut in wedges*

Blueberry muffins

- *250g plain flour*
- *200g brown sugar*
- *250g unsalted butter, softened*
- *4 eggs*
- *2 teaspoons baking powder*
- *150g fresh blueberries*
- *½ teaspoon of vanilla essence or pod*

Spinach and sweet potato tart

In a hot pan, sauté the spinach with some olive oil. Cover and simmer on medium heat for a few minutes. Meanwhile. in a mixing bowl, mash the cooked potatoes and season well. Add the beaten eggs, ricotta, parmesan and cooled spinach to the potatoes, and stir until all ingredients are well combined.

Grease a muffin baking tray with sunflower oil. Place the rolled pastry over the hollow cups and spoon the mixture inside. Repeat the process until all the filling is used. Cut the remaining pastry sheet in circles and cover the tarts. Brush the top with some milk or egg wash, and bake in a preheated oven 170°C for about 20-25 minutes until pies are golden.

Blueberry muffins

Preheat the oven to 180 Arrange twelve paper muffin cases on a baking tray. To make the muffins, beat the butter and sugar until pale and fluffy. Gradually add the eggs, beating well between additions. Sift the baking powder and flour together into the mixture. Mix in gently the blueberries and the vanilla essence.

Spoon the batter in the paper cases ⅔ full. Bake for 20 to 25 minutes, until the muffins are golden brown.

12

KUKU BLACK RICE WITH AVOCADO
* * *
GRAPES AND PEARS
* * *
YOGHURT POT CAKE

SERVES TWO LUNCHBOXES

Kuku black rice with avocado

This is a delicious take on the most classic of all the Persian kuku (frittata) recipes.

- vegetable oil
- one red onion, finely chopped
- 200g kale, stocks discarded and finely chopped
- 2 eggs, beaten
- 100g feta cheese, crumbled
- 100g black rice, cooked as per packet instructions
- a bunch of finely chopped parsley

Condiments

- 2 cups of grapes, deseeded and halved
- 2 pears, cleaned and quartered

Yoghurt cake

- 150g plain yoghurt
- 150ml flavourless vegetable oil
- 3 eggs
- 250g castor sugar
- a few drops of vanilla essence or pods
- 175g plain flour
- 75g corn flour

Kuku black rice with avocado

Heat a large saucepan over medium temperature. Pour in enough vegetable oil to coat the base of the pan and allow it to heat up. Then add the onion and fry gently for a few minutes, stirring from time to time until soft and cooked through. Add the kale, season with salt and pepper, and cook until the kale softens. Once cooked, take the pan off the heat and leave to cool.

Crack the eggs into a large mixing bowl and whisk. Add to the kale and onions, and heat until the egg mixture is cooked through. When the black rice is cooked as per packet instructions, drain and add to the pan with the egg, kale and onion. Stir until all the ingredients are well combined. Sprinkle the crumbs of feta cheese on top, and portion in a separate compartment of the lunchbox. In the compartment next to the rice, add chunky-chopped avocado and drizzle lemon or lime juice to avoid browning. Finally add a sprinkle of parsley over the rice and the avocado.

Yoghurt cake

Preheat the oven to 180°C and grease a ring mould baking tray using vegetable oil or baking spray. Separate the eggs and put the whites in one bowl and the yolks in another. Whisk the whites until you have a firm peak, and set aside.

Whisk together the pot of yoghurt, yolks and sugar until airy and light. Slowly add the vegetable oil while mixing. Add the vanilla extract and the zest of half a lemon, while still beating the mixture. Continue by adding the flour and the cornflour. When the batter is smooth and well combined, add dollops of whisked egg whites and fold them in with a spatula with the rest of the batter. Fill the prepared ring mould with the smooth soft batter until it comes right to the top. Bake in the oven for 30 to 35 minutes. When cooked, the sides will be coming away at the edges, and a cake tester will come out clean. Before serving, let the cake set in the tin for at least 30 minutes.

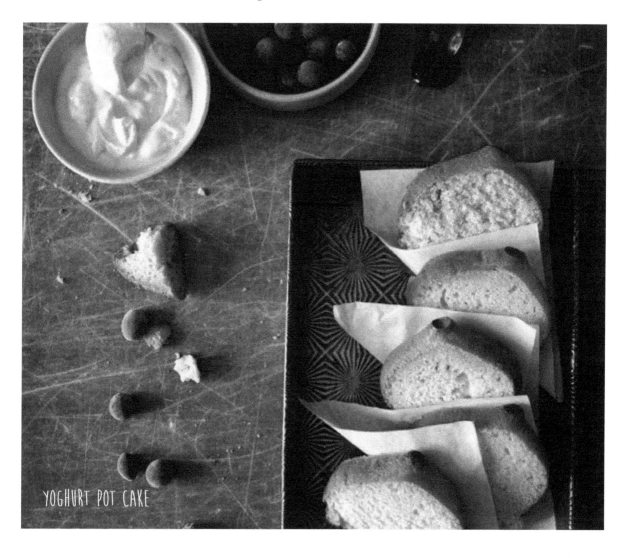

YOGHURT POT CAKE

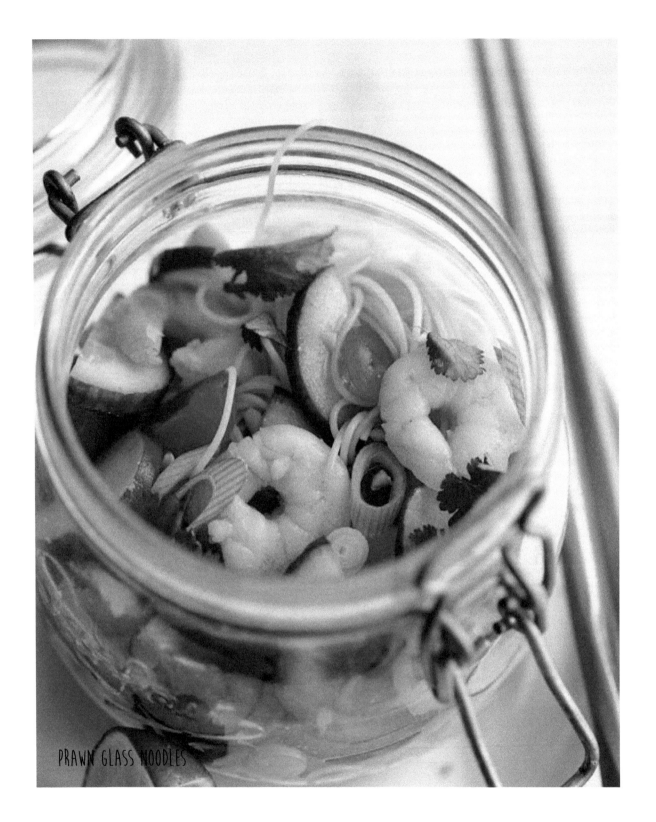

PRAWN GLASS NOODLES

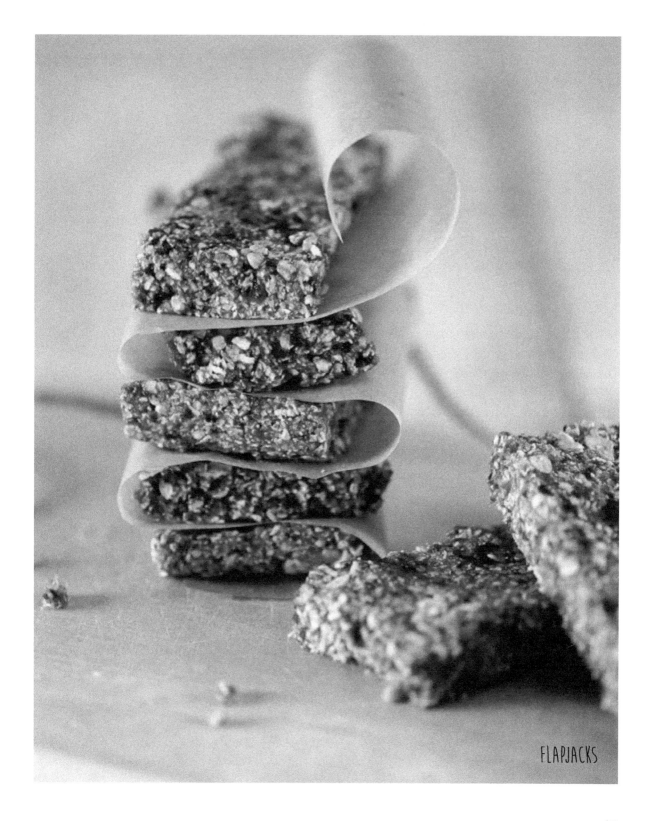

FLAPJACKS

13

PRAWN GLASS NOODLES
***
CITRUS AND POMEGRANATE
***
FLAPJACKS

SERVES TWO LUNCHBOXES

Prawn glass noodles

- *1 tablespoon sesame oil*
- *6 baby corn on the cob, sliced lengthwise*
- *1 red pepper, finely sliced*
- *300g small shrimp, cooked*
- *1 spring onion, finely chopped*
- *100g rice noodles, cooked (you may use any type of noodles)*
- *1 tablespoon sweet chilli*
- *a bunch fresh coriander, finely chopped*

Condiments

- *2 grapefruits, cleaned, deseeded and cut in wedges*
- *1 pomegranate, deseeded from its skin and shared between two lunchboxes*

Flapjacks

- *175g butter*
- *175g golden syrup*
- *175g muscovado sugar*
- *350g porridge oats*
- *zest of lemon, finely grated*
- *1 teaspoon grated fresh ginger*

Prawn glass noodles

Heat the wok or a flying pan on high temperature, and cook the spring onion, red pepper and corn over high heat until vegetables are softened but still crunchy. Remove from the heat and allow to cool. When the vegetables have cooled, add the cooked noodles, cooked shrimps, sweet chilli and chopped coriander. Stir well until all the flavours are evenly combined.

Flapjacks

Preheat the oven to 150. Line a baking tray with baking paper. Melt the butter gently, add the golden syrup and sugar to the butter and let it dissolve on low heat. When the emulsion has completely dissolved, remove from the heat and mix with the oats, lemon zest and ginger. Combine well until the oats are evenly coated with the liquid butter mixture. Pack the mixture into the baking tray and squash down to consolidate the ingredients. Bake in a preheated oven for 40 minutes.

Once cooked, remove from the oven. Leave to cool for 20 minutes, then turn out on a chopping board and cut into squares.

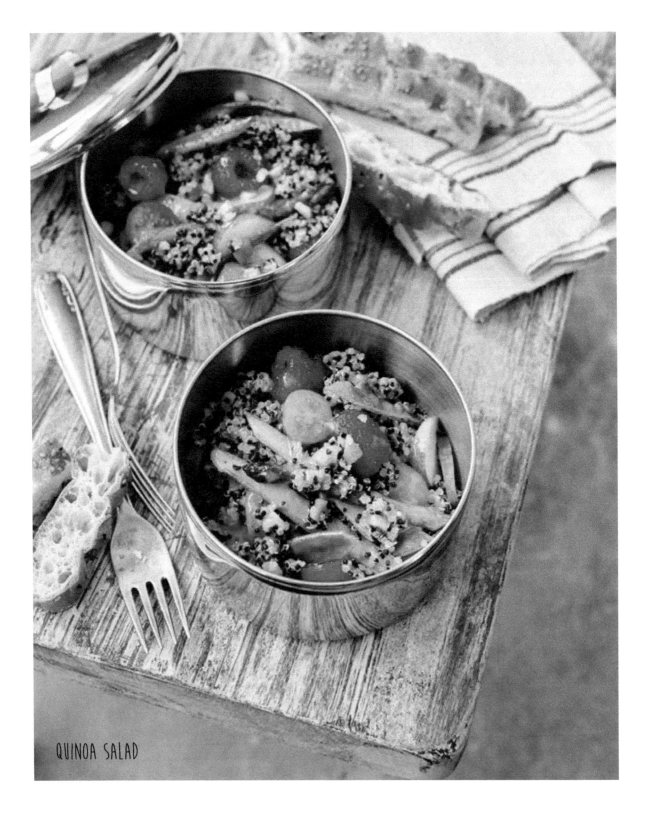

QUINOA SALAD

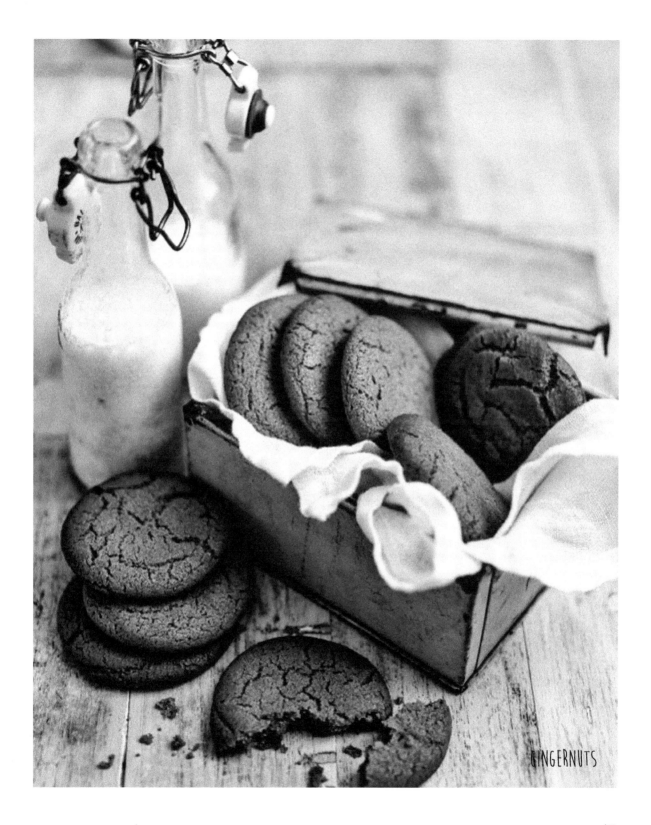

GINGERNUTS

14

QUINOA SALAD
* * *
FANCY CHEESE PLATTER
* * *
GINGERNUTS

SERVES TWO LUNCHBOXES

Quinoa salad

- *100g quinoa, cooked as per packet instructions*
- *50g chick peas, cooked*
- *a handful of dried cranberries*
- *a bunch of coriander leaves, chopped finely*
- *1 avocado, cut in chunks*

Dressing

- *1 tablespoon sesame oil*
- *1 tablespoon soy sauce*
- *½ lemon juice*

Mix all the ingredients together until well combined and smooth.

Fancy cheese platter

- *1 apple, cut in chunks*
- *1 pear, cut in chunks*
- *10 green grapes*
- *10 red grapes*
- *short kebab sticks*
- *1 cube of parmigiano, grana, manchego and comte*

You can vary the cheese selection for a more adventurous tasting experience or use only one type of a preferred cheese.

The fruit should be chopped in small chunks and arranged in each kebab stick. Children will enjoy arranging the fruits in a particular pattern.

Gingernuts

- *350g of self-raising flour*
- *200g castor sugar*
- *1 teaspoon finely grated fresh ginger*
- *1 teaspoon bicarbonate of soda*
- *125g butter*
- *75g golden syrup*
- *1 egg, beaten*
- *1 teaspoon grated orange rind*

Makes thirty biscuits. The uncooked batter is suitable to freeze.

Quinoa salad

Mix all the ingredients together except for the avocado, and drizzle over ¾ of the dressing. In a small bowl, add the chopped avocado and the rest of the dressing. Combine well and place in a separate compartment of the lunchbox next to the quinoa salad.

Gingernuts

Lightly grease a few baking trays and line with baking paper. Sieve the flour, sugar and bicarbonate of soda into a large mixing bowl.

Heat the butter and the golden syrup together in a saucepan over a very low heat until the butter has melted. Leave the butter mixture to cool slightly, then pour over the dry ingredients.

Add the egg, the fresh ginger and the orange rind, and mix thoroughly. Using your hands, carefully shape the dough into thirty even-sized balls.

Place the balls well apart on the prepared baking tray. Flatten them slightly with your fingers for the balls to resemble cookies. Bake in a preheated oven at 160 for 15 to 20 minutes. Before transferring them, let them cool completely.

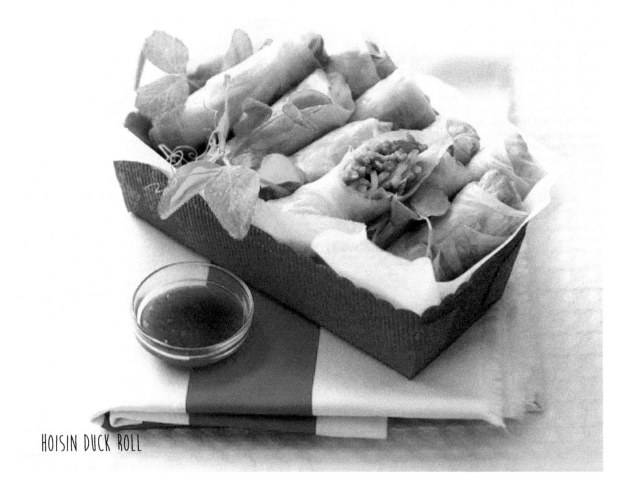

HOISIN DUCK ROLL

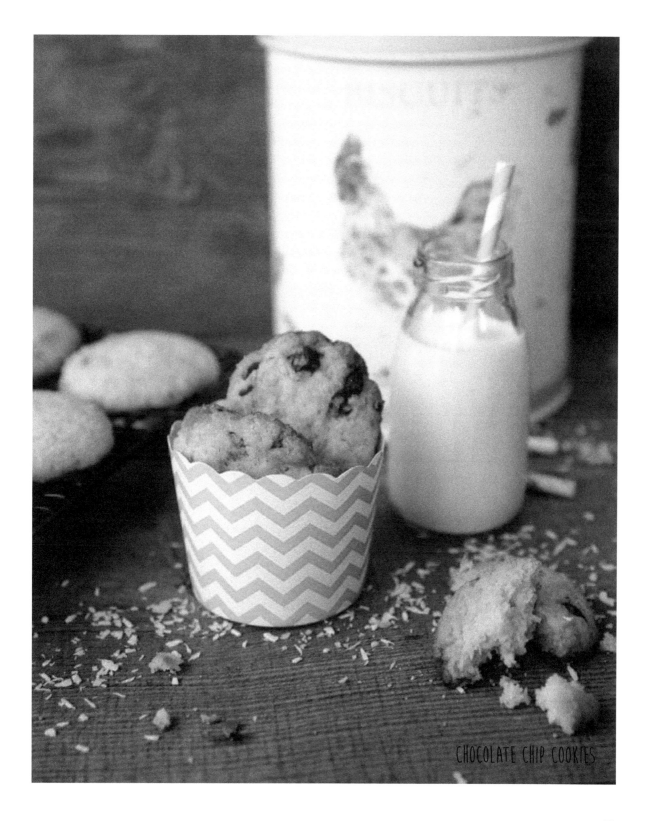

CHOCOLATE CHIP COOKIES

15

HOISIN DUCK ROLL
❊ ❊ ❊
WINTER MACEDONIA
❊ ❊ ❊
CHOCOLATE CHIP COOKIES

Hoisin duck roll

- *8 rice paper wrappers*
- *20g hoisin sauce*
- *2 spring onions, cut lengthwise very thinly*
- *½ cucumber, peeled and deseeded, and cut lengthwise very thinly*
- *1 handful of baby spinach leaves for each lunchbox*
- *shredded roasted duck meat*

This recipe is a real lunchbox treat. It is an ideal preparation after a Sunday roast or an Asian take out. You do not have to roast a whole duck. There are plenty of outlets that offer duck breast or duck legs alone.

Winter macedonia

- *1 banana*
- *2 kiwis*
- *juice of half an orange*
- *a handful of pomegranate*

Chop the banana and the kiwi in same-size chunks. Mix in a bowl, gently pouring over the orange juice. Place neatly in a separate compartment of the lunchbox and sprinkle a handful of pomegranate seeds.

Double choc chip cookies

- *110g butter, softened*
- *200g soft light brown sugar*
- *1 egg*
- *seeds of 1 vanilla pod or 2 drops of vanilla extract*
- *165g plain flour*
- *pinch of salt*
- *½ teaspoon baking powder*
- *½ teaspoon bicarbonate of soda*
- *30g cocoa powder*
- *100g good-quality milk chocolate chips*
- *100g good-quality dark chocolate chips*

Hoisin duck roll

Half fill a bowl with cold water. Submerge a rice paper until soft and pliable but not completely soggy. Lay on a chopping board and spread the hoisin sauce over half the wrap. Place the baby spinach leaves over the spread. Then add the duck, onion and cucumber. Roll up by bringing the bottom and the top edge of the wrapper over the filling. Fold one side over and roll tightly.

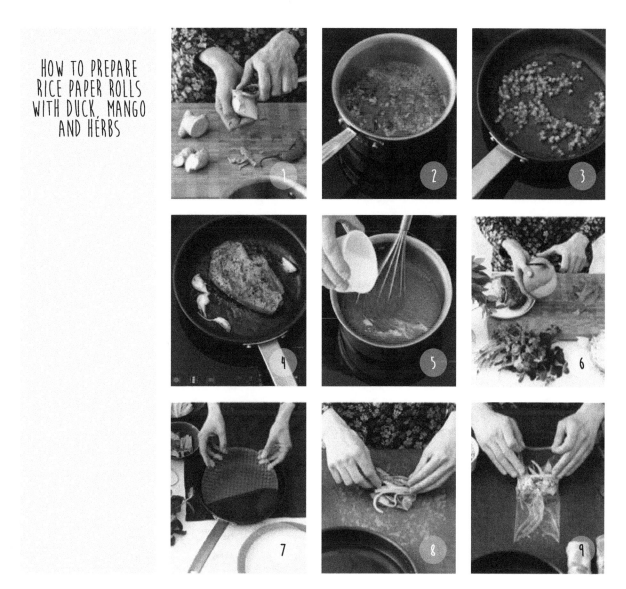

Double choc chip cookies

Preheat the oven at 180. Line two large baking trays with baking paper. Put the butter and the sugar in a large bowl and cream together until combined. Stir in the egg and vanilla and mix well until smooth. Add the flour, salt, baking powder, bicarbonate of soda and cocoa powder, and mix until the dough is uniform. Add the chocolate chips and fold with a wooden spoon or spatula.

Divide the mixture into balls and space them on the prepared baking tray and flatten slightly with your fingers. Bake for 10 to 12 minutes until the cookies crack on the top but are still soft in texture.

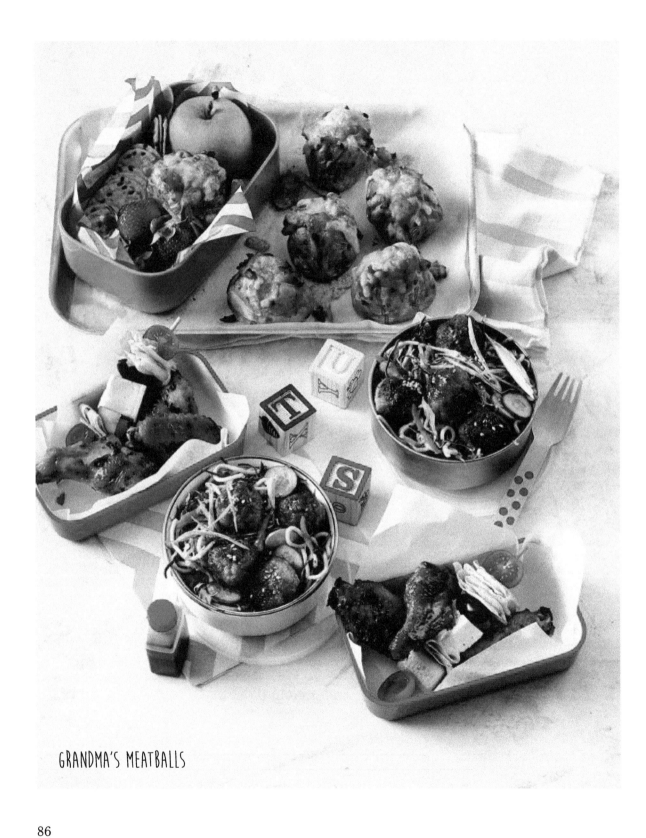

GRANDMA'S MEATBALLS

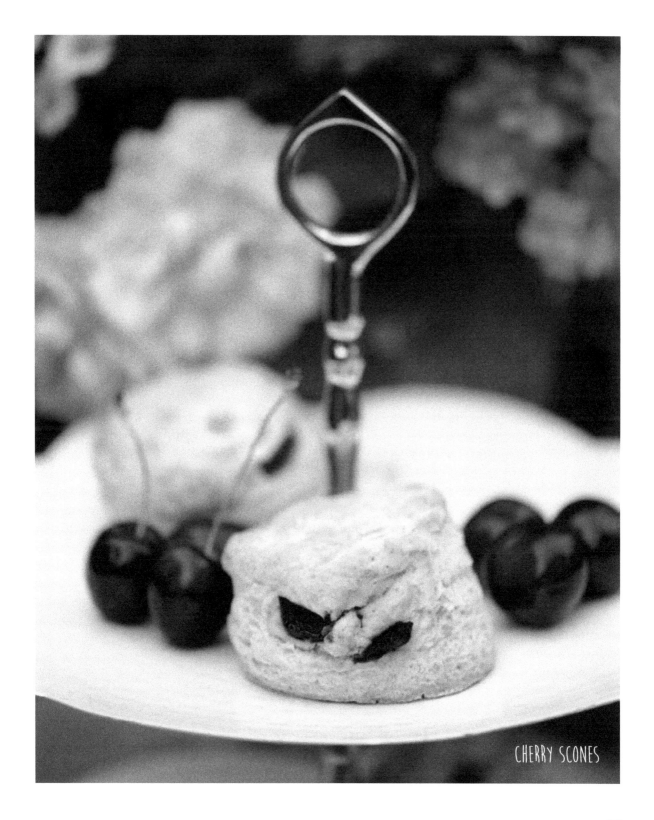

CHERRY SCONES

16

GRANDMA'S MEATBALLS
***
AUTUMN VEGETABLES
***
CHERRY SCONES

SERVES TWO LUNCHBOXES

Grandma's meatballs

- *1 kg minced beef*
- *1 onion, finely chopped*
- *olive oil*
- *3 tablespoons red wine vinegar*
- *1 clove garlic, crushed finely*
- *90g panko breadcrumbs*
- *a bunch of fresh mint*
- *a bunch of fresh parsley*
- *1 egg*

Cherry scones

- *225g self-raising flour*
- *1 tablespoon castor sugar*
- *pinch of salt*
- *75g butter, cut into small pieces*
- *40g candied cherries*
- *40g sultanas*
- *1 egg, beaten*
- *50ml milk*

Autumn vegetables

- *100g green beans, tips cut off and halved*
- *2 large potatoes, peeled, sliced and boiled*
- *olive oil*
- *juice of a half a lemon*
- *oregano*

Before arranging the vegetables in the lunchbox, season them well with olive oil, lemon juice, oregano, and salt and pepper, and season well.

Condiments

- *a handful of banana chips for each lunchbox*
- *2 pots of yoghurt of your choice*

Grandma's meatballs

Put all the ingredients for the meatballs, except the olive oil, in a large bowl and use your hands to mix them well together. Cover and leave to rest in the refrigerator for an hour. Meanwhile, preheat the oven to 200°C. Roll the meatball mixture directly from the refrigerator into small balls.

Place the meatball on a greased and lined baking tray. Drizzle with olive oil and bake for around ten minutes. Remove from the oven and leave them to rest for a few minutes.

Cherry scones

Lightly grease a baking tray and line with baking paper. Sieve the flour, sugar and salt into a mixing bowl and rub in the butter with your fingers until the scone mixture resembles breadcrumbs.

Stir in the candied cherries, sultanas and egg. Reserve one tablespoon of the milk for glazing, then add the remainder to the mixture. Mix together to form a soft dough.

On a lightly floured surface, roll out the dough to a thickness of 2 cm. Using a round cutter, cut out eight scones. Place the scones onto a baking tray and brush with the reserved milk. Bake in a preheated oven at 220°C for around ten minutes, until the scones are golden brown.

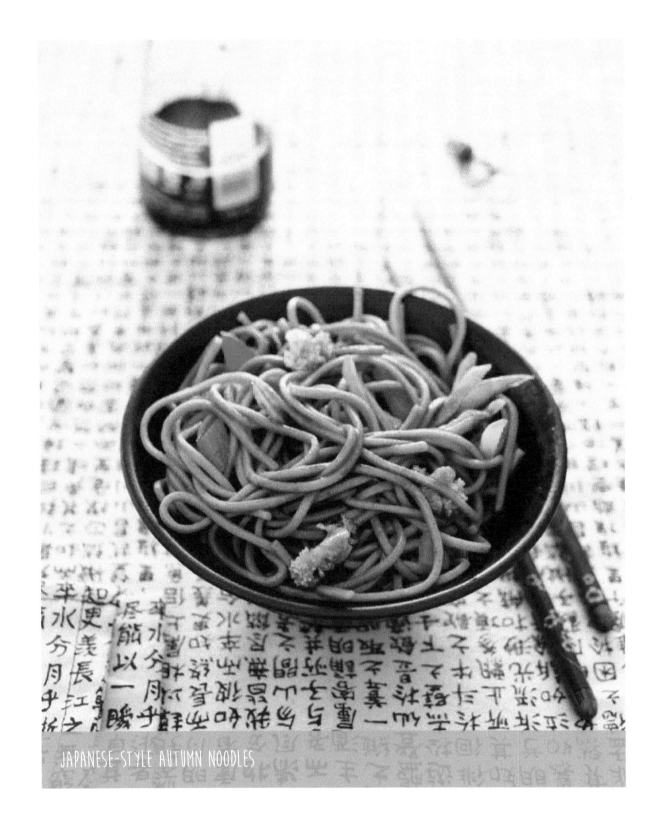

JAPANESE-STYLE AUTUMN NOODLES

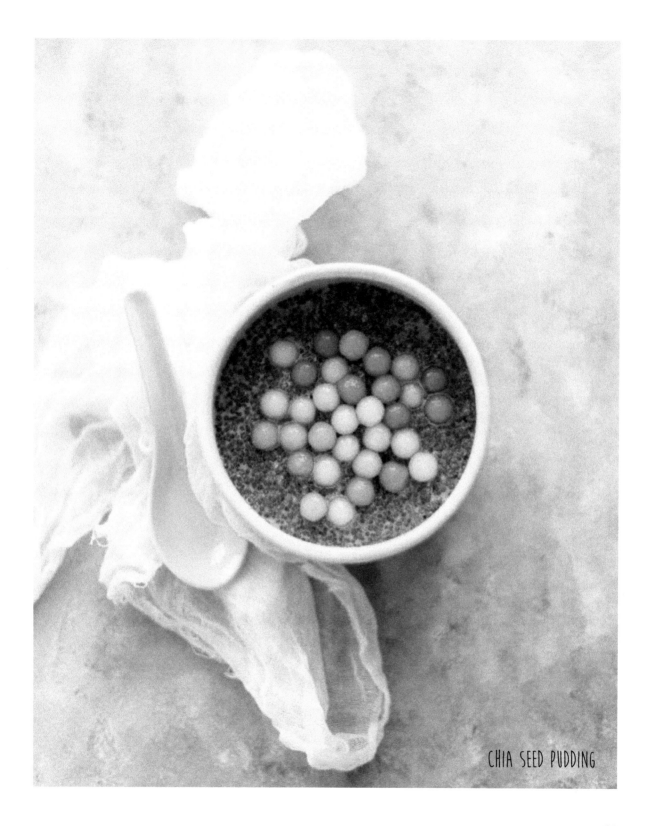

CHIA SEED PUDDING

17

JAPANESE-STYLE AUTUMN NOODLES
✱ ✱ ✱
DATES AND CITRUS MIX
✱ ✱ ✱
CHIA SEED PUDDING

SERVES TWO LUNCHBOXES

Japanese-style autumn noodles

- *100g soba noodles, cooked as per packet instructions*
- *5 Brussels sprouts, stalks removed, quartered*
- *5 small broccoli florets, halved*
- *seaweed, roughly torn*
- *1 tablespoon sesame oil*
- *1 tablespoon soy sauce*
- *1 teaspoon clear honey*
- *a handful of mixed sesame seeds, toasted*

Condiments

- *8 good-quality dates*
- *2 whole tangerines or clementines*

Chia Pudding

- *1 banana*
- *½ teaspoon vanilla essence*
- *1 cup coconut milk*
- *½ cup black chia seeds*

Chia Pudding

Using an electric mixer, blend the coconut milk, banana and vanilla. When smooth, add the chia seeds and stir well with a spatula. Take care not to crush the seeds. Cover and leave in the blender or tip in a glass jar. Refrigerate overnight and place in a small compartment of the lunchbox when needed.

Japanese-style autumn noodles

Stir-fry the Brussels sprouts and the broccoli in the sesame oil on high heat until the vegetables are softened but still crunchy. Switch off the heat and add the cooked noodles, soy sauce, crushed seaweed, clear honey and sesame oil. Toss the noodles well until all the ingredients are combined. Before you arrange in the lunchbox, let the noodles cool to absorb all the flavours. Garnish with toasted sesame seeds.

18

AVOCADO WRAP
* * *
AUTUMN SNACKS
* * *
CARAWAY BISCUITS

SERVES TWO LUNCHBOXES

Avocado wrap

- *2 tortilla wraps*
- *½ cup ricotta*
- *1 tablespoon pesto*
- *a handful of baby spinach leaves*
- *4 slices tomatoes*
- *a bunch of basil, torn roughly*
- *1 avocado, shredded hard matured*
- *Italian pecorino or parmesan cheese*

Easy homemade pesto

- *2 tablespoons mixed pumpkin, sesame and sunflower seeds*
- *1 cup packed fresh basil*
- *juice of 1 lemon*
- *¼ cup olive oil to start (add if necessary)*

Blend all the pesto ingredients until smooth. Add oil if necessary. Pour over the vegetable salad and stir until all the ingredients are evenly combined.

Avocado wrap

In a mixing bowl, crush the avocado until mashed. Add the pesto and the ricotta and season well with salt and pepper. Spread the mixture over the tortilla and top with spinach and tomato slices. Sprinkle with basil leaves and shredded cheese. Fold the edges to secure the ingredients and roll tightly. Serve halved or quartered in a separate compartment of the lunchbox.

Autumn snacks

- *2 oranges, cut in supremes*
- *2 hard-boiled eggs*
- *shredded seaweed*
- *a handful of mixed luxury dried fruit (pineapple, papaya, raisins)*

Halve the hard-boiled eggs and sprinkle with the shredded seaweed.

Caraway biscuits

- *225g all-purpose flour*
- *pinch of salt*
- *100g butter, cut in small pieces*
- *225g castor sugar*
- *1 egg, beaten*
- *2 tablespoons caraway seeds*

Grease a few baking trays and line them with baking paper. Sieve the flour and salt into a mixing bowl. Rub the butter with your fingers until the mixture resembles fine breadcrumbs. Stir in the castor sugar.

Reserve a tablespoon of egg mixture for brushing the top of the biscuits. Add the rest of the egg to the mixture along with the caraway seeds and combine until a soft dough forms.

On a lightly-floured surface, roll the biscuit dough until quite thin. With a round cutter, cut out five-centimetre diameter biscuits and transfer on a prepared baking tray. Bake in a preheated oven at 160 for around 15 minutes until lightly golden and crisp.

Leave the biscuits to cool before placing in the lunchbox or an airtight container.

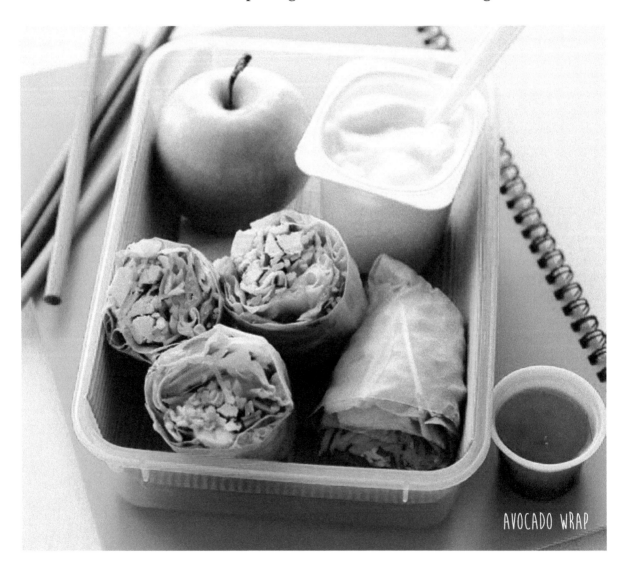

AVOCADO WRAP

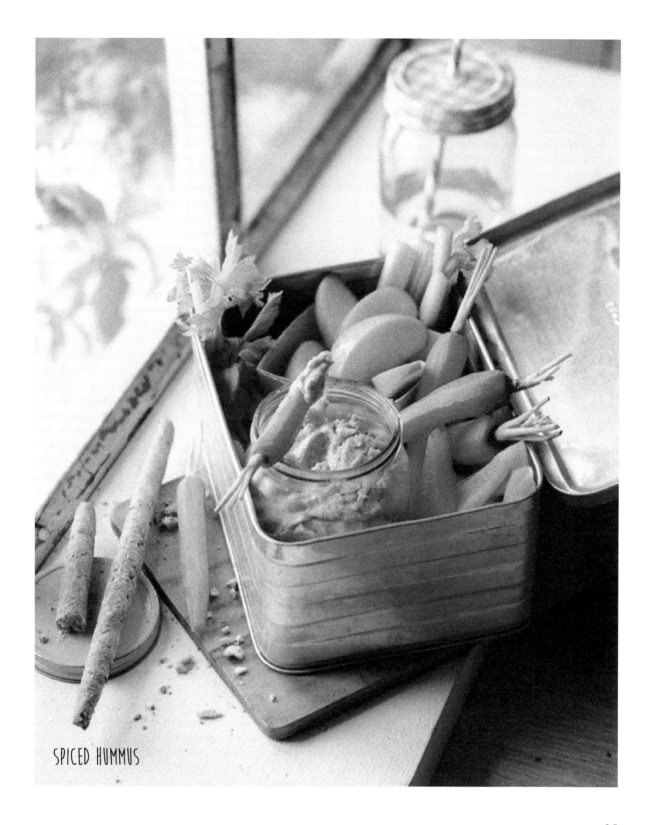

SPICED HUMMUS

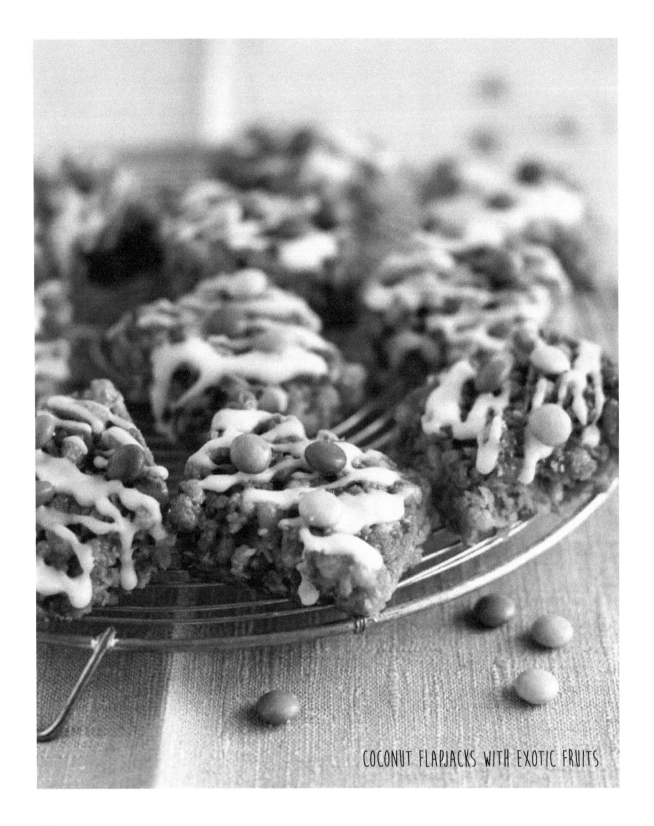

COCONUT FLAPJACKS WITH EXOTIC FRUITS

19

GIANT COUSCOUS SALAD
**
SPICED HUMMUS AND CARROTS
**
COCONUT FLAPJACKS WITH EXOTIC FRUITS

SERVES TWO LUNCHBOXES

Giant couscous salad

- *100g giant couscous, cooked as per packet instructions*
- *olive oil*
- *½ red pepper, diced finely*
- *½ yellow pepper, diced finely*
- *a bunch of dill, finely chopped*
- *a bunch of parsley, finely chopped*
- *1 tablespoon clear honey*
- *1 tablespoon balsamic vinegar*

Spiced hummus

- *200g chickpeas, cooked as per packet instructions*
- *fresh turmeric, finely grated*
- *1 clove garlic*
- *1 teaspoon cumin seeds, toasted and crushed*
- *juice and zest of 1 lemon*
- *4 teaspoons tahini*
- *olive oil*

Coconut flapjacks

- *200g butter*
- *200g demerara sugar*
- *2 tablespoons golden syrup*
- *275g porridge oats*
- *100g desiccated coconut*
- *75g dried pineapple or currants*

Condiments

- *2 carrots, peeled and cut in strips lengthwise*
- *1 mango, peeled, deboned and sliced*
- *a handful of raspberries*

Giant couscous salad

Boil the couscous according to packet instructions. When cooked, drain and rinse thoroughly under cold water until completely cool. Drain and set aside. Heat the olive oil in a saucepan over medium heat. Add peppers, and sauté until soft and browned at the edges. Set aside to cool.

In a large mixing bowl add couscous, cooked peppers and all the pan juices, parsley, dill, honey and balsamic vinegar. Stir well until all ingredients are evenly combined.

Spiced hummus

Use a food processor to blitz the chickpeas with olive oil and lemon juice till smooth. Pour some of the water used to cook chick peas, if necessary. Add the fresh turmeric, crushed cumin seeds, lemon zest and tahini, and season well. Blend until completely combined and smooth.

Coconut flapjack

Lightly grease a baking tray and line with baking paper. Heat the butter, sugar and golden syrup in a saucepan until just melted over low heat. Stir in oats and dried fruit and stir until evenly combined.

Spread the mixture on the prepared baking tray and press down to consolidate the ingredients. Use a palette knife to level before baking in a preheated oven at 170 for about 30 minutes.

Remove from the oven and leave it to cool completely in its tray. Cut the mixture into squares using a sharp knife.

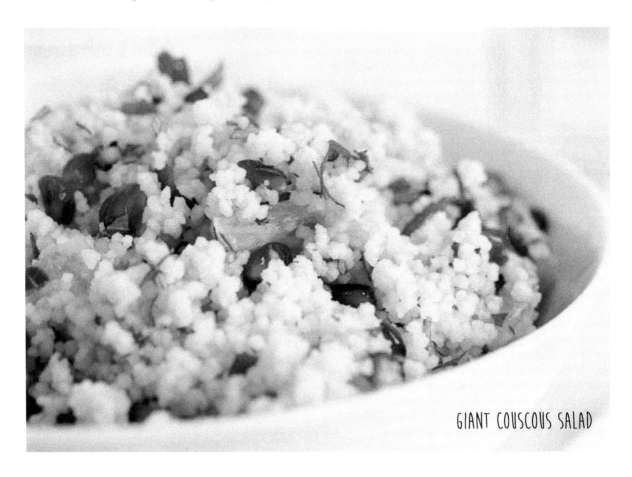

GIANT COUSCOUS SALAD

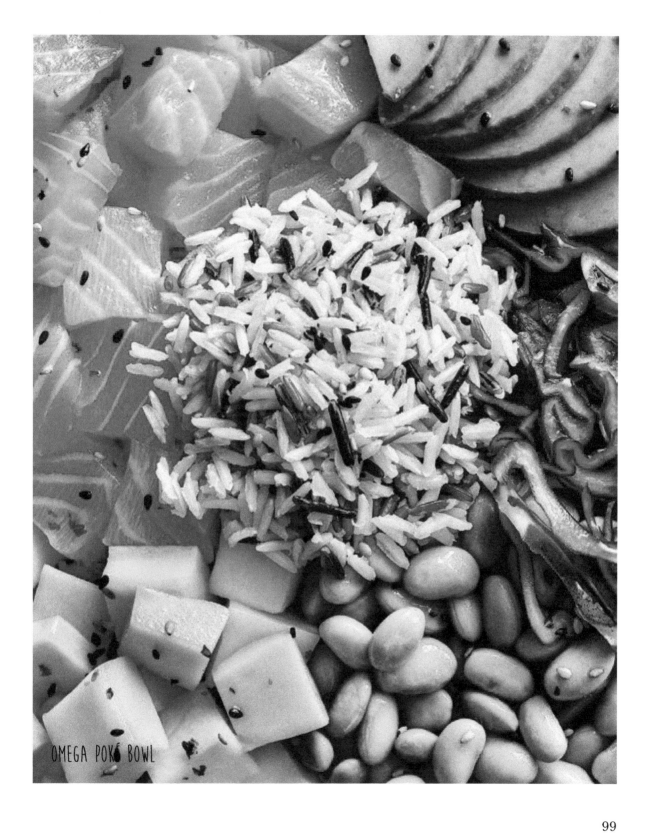

OMEGA POKÉ BOWL

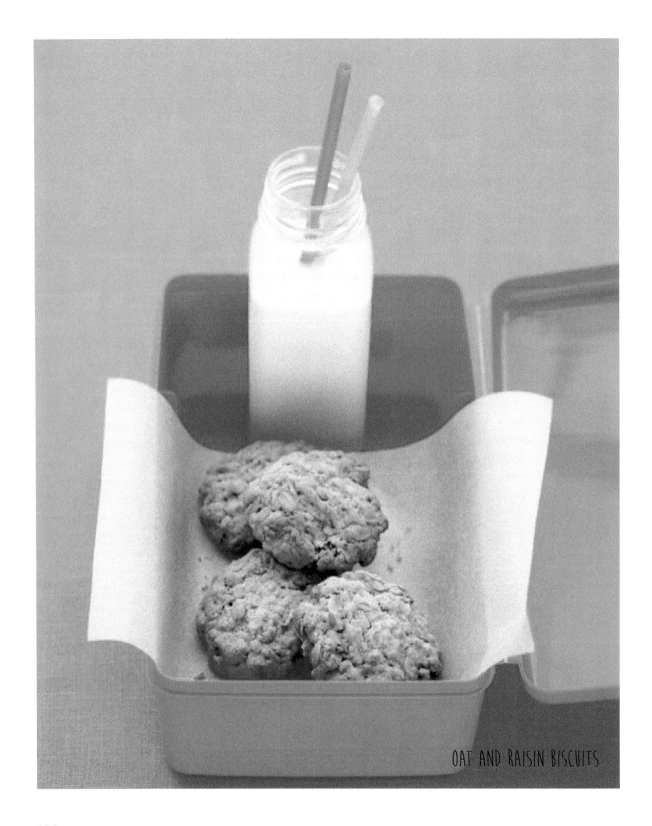

OAT AND RAISIN BISCUITS

20

OMEGA POKÉ BOWL
OAT AND RAISIN BISCUITS

SERVES TWO LUNCHBOXES

Omega poké bowl

- 100g basmati rice, cooked as per packet instructions
- 200g cooked salmon
- ½ cup teriyaki sauce
- edamame beans
- 1 tomato, cut in chunks
- 2 grated carrots
- ½ cucumber, finely sliced
- seaweed flakes
- 1 avocado, peeled, deboned and finely sliced

Rice dressing

- 1 tablespoon soy sauce
- 1 tablespoon sesame oil

Condiments

- 1 pear
- 2 kiwis
- a handful of blueberries for each lunchbox

Oat and raisin biscuits

- 50g butter
- 125g castor sugar
- 1 egg, beaten
- 50g all-purpose flour
- ½ teaspoon salt
- ½ teaspoon baking powder
- 175g porridge oats
- 125g raisins
- 2 tablespoons sesame seeds

Omega poké bowl

Cook the basmati rice according to its packet instructions. Drain and tip in a mixing bowl, add the soy sauce and the sesame oil and stir well with a fork until the rice is well coated and rice grains are separated. Meanwhile, cook the salmon fillet, place the cleaned fish on a lined baking tray and pour over the teriyaki sauce. Bake for ten minutes in a preheated oven at 160. When cooked, set aside to cool. Then cut in squares with a sharp knife.

Place the rice in a lunchbox compartment, covering the whole surface. Start constructing your poké bowl by placing the remaining ingredients over the rice, neatly next to one another.

Oat and raisin biscuits

Lightly grease two baking trays and line with baking paper. In a large mixing bowl, cream together the butter and the sugar until light and fluffy. Add the beaten egg gradually until well combined.

Sieve the flour, salt and baking powder into the creamed mixture. Mix well, then add the oats, raisins, and sesame seeds and mix together thoroughly.

Place spoonfuls of the mixture well apart on the prepared baking trays and flatten them slightly with the back of a spoon. Bake in a preheated oven at 180 for about 15 minutes. Leave the biscuit to cool completely before serving or storing.

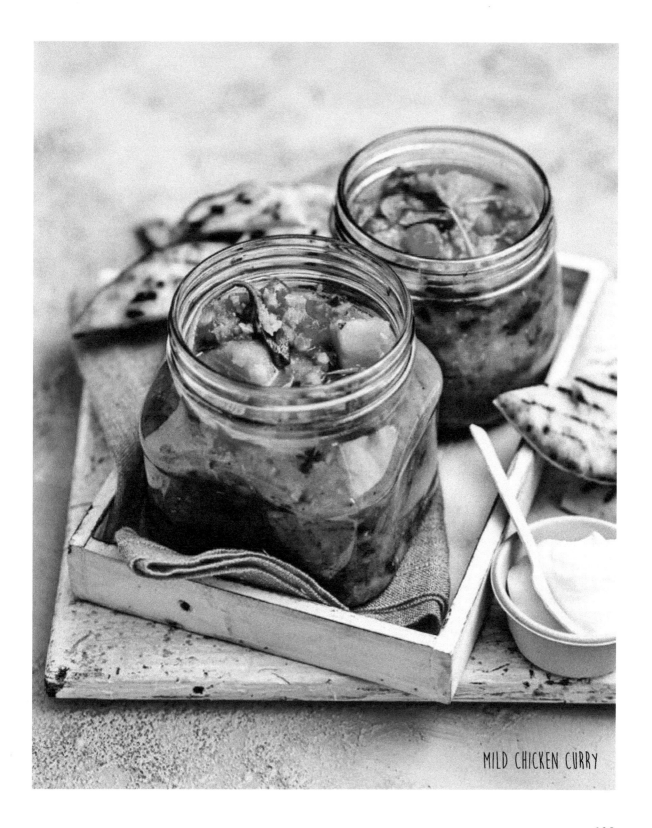

MILD CHICKEN CURRY

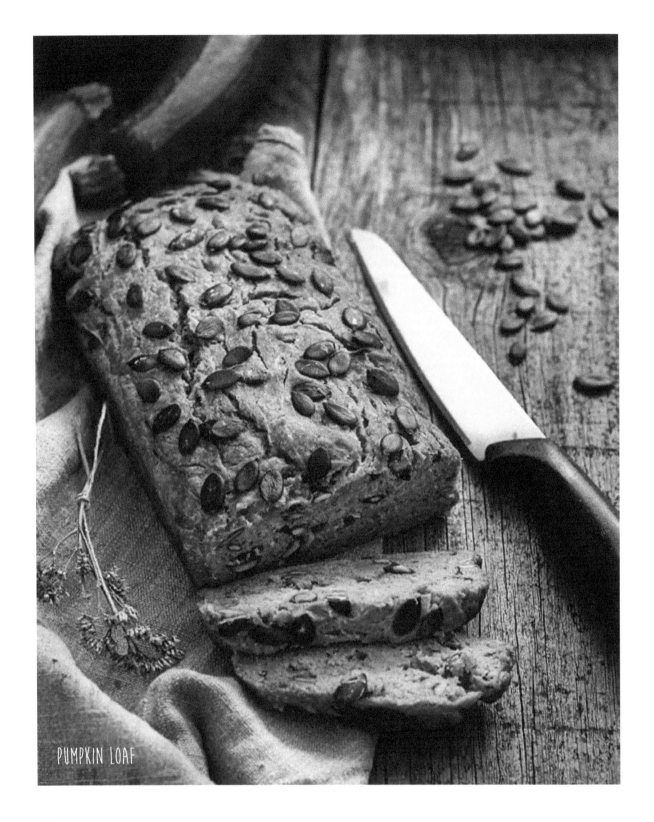

PUMPKIN LOAF

21

MILD CHICKEN CURRY
* * *
TOMATO AND MANGO SALAD
* * *
PUMPKIN LOAF

SERVES TWO LUNCHBOXES

Mild chicken curry

- *1 chicken breast*
- *1 cup of coconut milk*
- *1 teaspoon green curry-mild paste*
- *2 tablespoons finely chopped leeks*
- *vegetable oil*
- *100g basmati rice, cooked as per packet instructions*
- *a bunch of finely chopped coriander*

Condiments

- *2 pitta breads or naan breads, quartered*

Tomato and mango salad

- *2 small tomatoes, quartered*
- *1 mango, peeled, deboned and finely sliced*
- *a bunch of coriander, finely chopped*
- *caramelised onions (optional)*

Mix the mango, tomatoes and coriander and organise in a lunchbox compartment. Top with a spoonful of caramelised onion. To caramelise onions, heat a pan with some vegetable oil. Cook the onions until they are transparent and soft. Add two tablespoons of maple syrup and half a cup of water for every onion, and let the liquid reduce until gooey.

Pumpkin loaf

- *450g pumpkin flesh*
- *125g butter*
- *175g castor sugar*
- *2 eggs, beaten*
- *225g all-purpose flour, sifted*
- *1½ teaspoon baking powder*
- *½ teaspoon salt*
- *1 tablespoon ground allspice*
- *25g pumpkin seeds*

Mild chicken curry

Cook the rice following the instructions on its packet. Meanwhile, chop the chicken breast in very small cubes. Heat some oil in a pan and cook the chicken on a high flame until golden brown. Add the leeks, lower the heat and cook further until the leeks have softened and the chicken is cooked through.

In a separate sauce pan dissolve the curry paste and add the coconut milk. Simmer on low heat until paste has dissolved and coconut milk is reduced. Pour some of the liquid over the rice and stir with a fork to separate the rice grains. Tip the rest of the liquid in the pan and stir the chicken until coated with the curry sauce. Place the rice in a separate compartment of the lunchbox and the chicken next to it. Sprinkle finely-chopped coriander.

Pumpkin loaf

Grease a loaf tin with some vegetable oil and line the bottom with baking paper. Chop the pumpkin in large chunks. Wrap the pieces in foil and bake in a preheated oven at 200 for 30 to 40 minutes until tender. When cooked, set aside to cool completely. In a bowl, cream the butter and sugar together until light and fluffy. Add the eggs and soft pumpkin and mix until all the ingredients have been well combined. Fold the flour, baking powder, salt and mixed spice. Finally, gently fold in the pumpkin seeds and pour the mixture in the prepared baking loaf tin. Bake in a preheated oven at 160 for around one hour and a half, until a skewer inserted in the centre of the loaf comes out clean. Leave the loaf to cool completely before slicing.

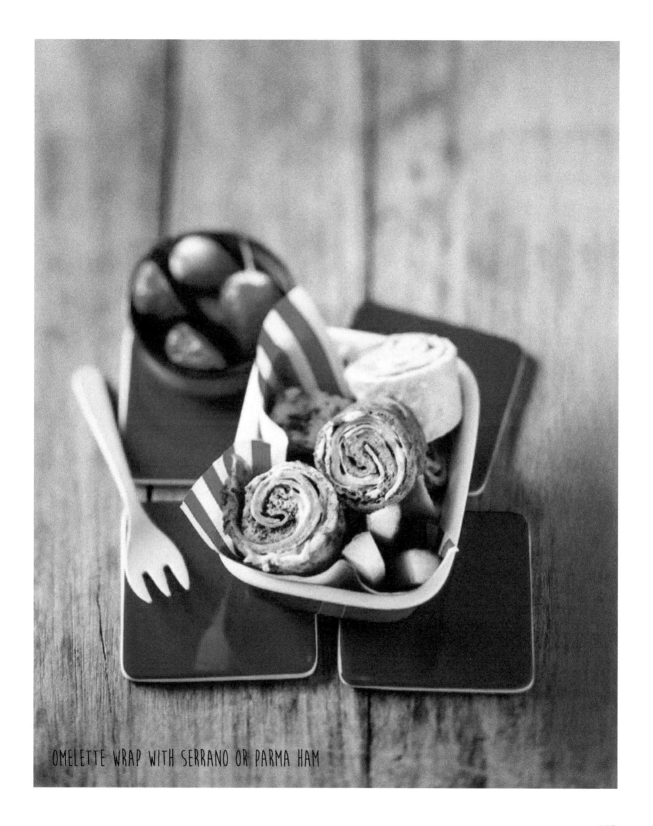

OMELETTE WRAP WITH SERRANO OR PARMA HAM

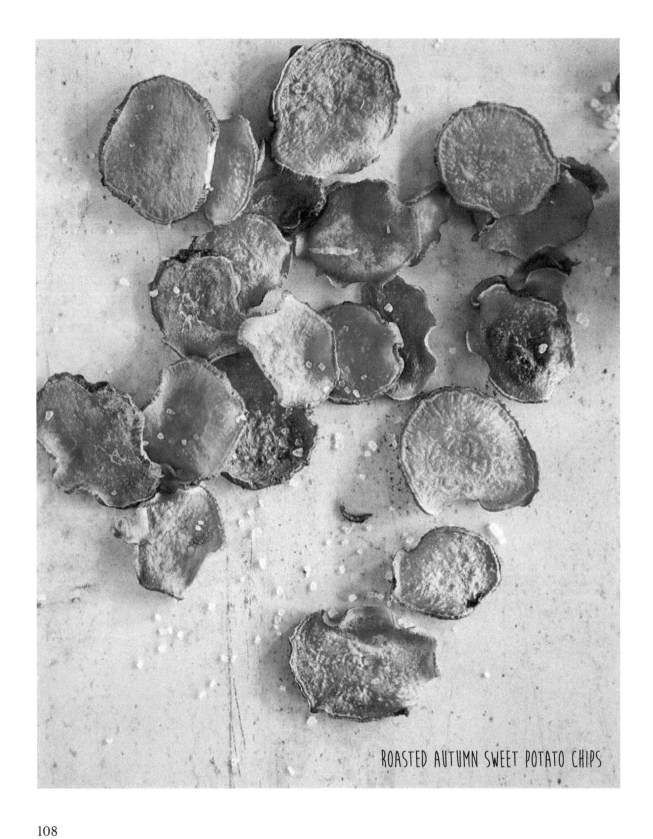

ROASTED AUTUMN SWEET POTATO CHIPS

22

OMELETTE WRAP WITH SERRANO OR PARMA HAM
☀ ☀ ☀
ROASTED AUTUMN SWEET POTATO CHIPS
☀ ☀ ☀
BANANA AND DATE LOAF

SERVES TWO LUNCHBOXES

Omelette wrap with Serrano or Parma ham

- *2 eggs*
- *1 tablespoon chives, finely chopped*
- *4 slices serrano or Parma ham*
- *a bunch of basil leaves, roughly torn*
- *2 corn soft tortillas*
- *1 tablespoon pesto*

Easy homemade pesto

- *2 tablespoons mixed pumpkin, sesame and sunflower seeds*
- *1 cup packed fresh basil*
- *juice of 1 lemon*
- *¼ cup olive oil to start (add if necessary)*

Blend all the pesto ingredients until smooth. Add oil if necessary. Pour over the vegetable salad and stir until all the ingredients are evenly combined.

Roasted autumn sweet potato chips

- *2 large sweet potatoes*
- *olive oil*
- *fresh rosemary*

Peel and cut the sweet potatoes in French fry shapes. Place in a mixing bowl and add rosemary and olive oil. Season well with salt and pepper, and toss until the potatoes are well coated. Tip the potatoes on a lined baking tray and bake in a preheated oven at 180 for about 45 minutes until crunchy on the outside but soft at the touch.

Condiments

- *2 cups of red grapes*
- *6 thin wedges of manchego or any hard cheese*
- *2 small tubs of Greek yoghurt*
- *drizzle of honey*

Banana and date loaf

- *225g self-raising flour*
- *100g butter, cut in small cubes*
- *75g castor sugar*
- *125g dates, stoned and chopped*
- *2 bananas, roughly mashed*
- *2 eggs*
- *2 tablespoons of honey*

Omelette wrap with Serrano or Parma ham

In a mixing bowl, add the eggs, the basil and the chives, and season well with salt and pepper. Stir vigorously until the mixture is light and fluffy. Cook the omelette in a hot pan until golden and crispy. Set aside to cool.

Spread the tortillas with a thin layer of pesto, place half of the omelette over one tortilla. Cover with the ham slices. Fold the bottom and the top edge over the ingredients and roll to seal the filling. Halve or quarter and place in a lunchbox compartment.

Banana and date loaf

Grease a loaf tin and line with baking paper. Sieve the flour into a mixing bowl. Rub the butter into the flour with your fingertips until the mixture resembles fine breadcrumbs. Stir in the sugar, the chopped dates, the beaten eggs, and the honey into the dry ingredients. Mix together to form a soft dropping consistency. Spoon the mixture into the prepared tin, level the surface with a spatula and bake in a preheated oven at 160 for about an hour, until the surface is golden and a skewer inserted in the middle of the loaf comes out clean. Leave the loaf to cool completely before slicing.

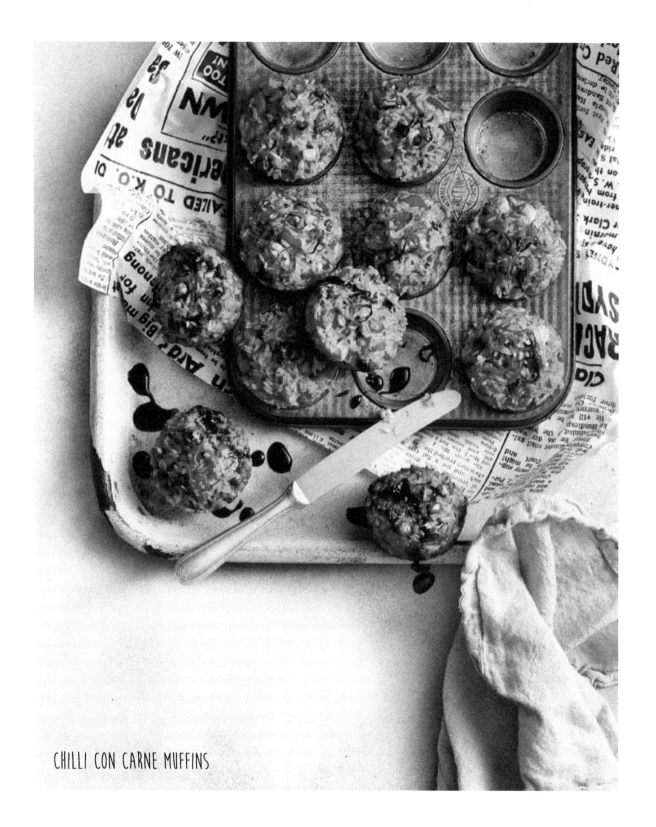

CHILLI CON CARNE MUFFINS

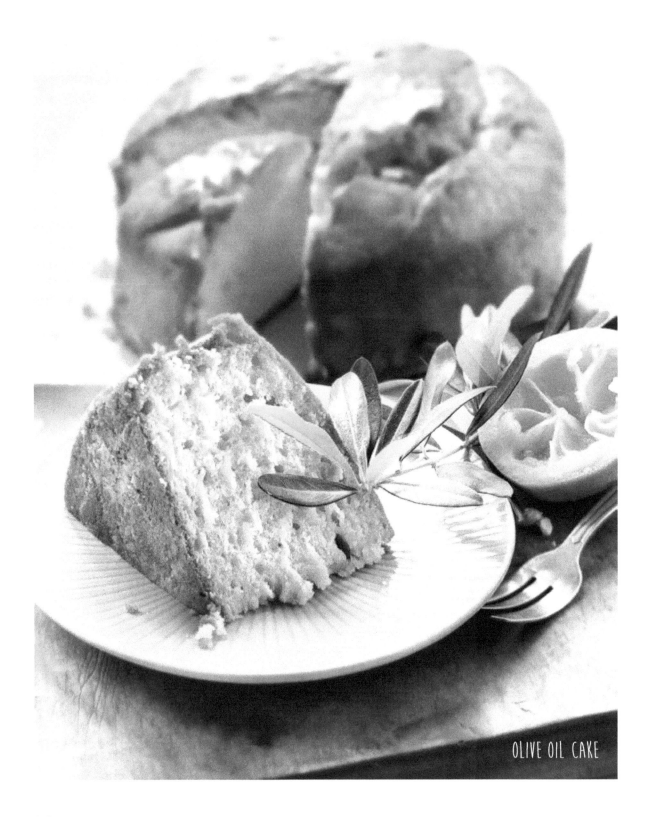

OLIVE OIL CAKE

23

CHILLI CON CARNE MUFFINS WITH MEXICAN CHUNKY SALSA
* * *
OLIVE OIL CAKE
* * *
PINEAPPLE SALAD

SERVES TWO LUNCHBOXES

Chilli con carne muffins

- *100g lean beef mince*
- *100g red kidney beans*
- *1 cup tomato pulp*
- *1 cup mix, finely chopped onion, celery and carrot*
- *olive oil*
- *½ teaspoon honey*
- *a bunch of finely chopped parsley*
- *100g long grain rice*
- *2 eggs, beaten*

Condiments

- *½ pineapple, cut in wedges*
- *2 red peppers, deseeded and cut in sticks lengthwise*
- *1 avocado, peeled, deboned and cut in slices lengthwise*

Olive oil cake

- *nonstick cooking spray*
- *200g light brown sugar*
- *zest of 1 orange*
- *zest of 1 lemon*
- *120ml olive oil*
- *3 large eggs, at room temperature*
- *2 tablespoons fresh-squeezed orange or lemon juice*
- *1 teaspoon pure vanilla extract*
- *155g whole-wheat flour*
- *1 teaspoon baking powder*
- *½ teaspoon fine sea salt*

Chilli con carne muffins

Grease a muffin baking tray and line with individual cupcake baking paper cups. Boil the rice as per packet instructions. In the meantime, cook the chilli con carne by frying the onion, celery and carrots in olive oil on high heat. When the vegetables are softened, add the meat and beans and cook through. Finally, add the tomato pulp and simmer on low heat till all the liquids have reduced and the sauce is dense.

Let the sauce cool for ten minutes, then add the rice and the beaten eggs. Mix well till all the ingredients are well combined. Spoon the mixture in the cupcake paper and bake in a preheated oven at 160 for about 20 minutes. The rice will look crunchy on the outside and will form a firm mould.

Olive oil cake

Preheat the oven to 180 . Lightly grease a loaf pan with nonstick spray. Mix the brown sugar, orange and lemon zests together in a medium bowl until well combined. Stir in the oil. Add the eggs one at a time, whisking in each one well before adding the next. Whisk in the juice and vanilla.

Stir together the whole-wheat flour, baking powder and the salt in a small bowl. Add the dry ingredients to the wet and mix with a rubber spatula just until incorporated. Pour the batter into the prepared pan and spread evenly.

Bake for 40 to 45 minutes until a toothpick inserted into the centre of the loaf comes out clean. Cool the cake in the pan for 15 minutes, then remove from the pan and cool completely on a rack before slicing and serving.

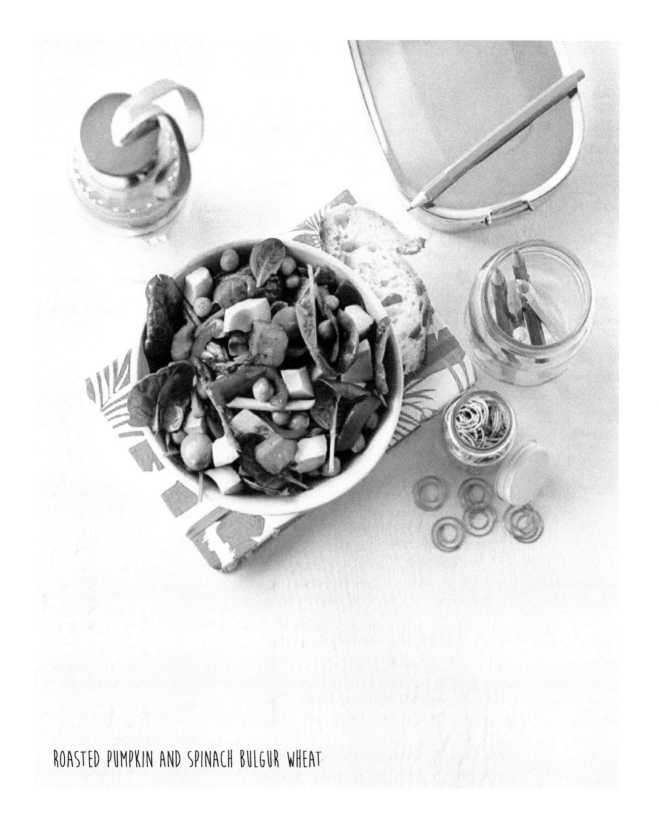

ROASTED PUMPKIN AND SPINACH BULGUR WHEAT

SERVES TWO LUNCHBOXES

Roasted, pumpkin and spinach bulgur wheat

- *200g pumpkin, roasted*
- *200g cooked spinach*
- *100g bulgur wheat, cooked as per packet instructions*
- *50g currants*
- *a bunch of coriander leaves, finely chopped*
- *olive oil*
- *½ tablespoon balsamic vinegar*
- *caramelised onion*

Carmelised onion

Mix the mango, tomatoes and coriander and organise in a lunchbox compartment. Top with a spoonful of caramelised onion. To caramelise onions, heat a pan with some vegetable oil. Cook the onions until they are transparent and soft. Add two tablespoons of maple syrup and half a cup of water for every onion, and let the liquid reduce until gooey.

Condiments

- *2 apples, peeled, cleaned and quartered*
- *a handful of pomegranates*
- *8 dried apricots*
- *8 dates*
- *80g feta cheese, cubed, drizzled with honey and sprinkled with oregano*

Roasted pumpkin and spinach bulgur wheat

This dish is served as a poké bowl construction. First cook the bulgur wheat as instructed on its packet. Dress the cooked wheat with olive oil, balsamic vinegar, currants and chopped coriander. Mix well and place in the lunchbox, covering the surface. Assemble the pumpkin, spinach and caramelised onion over the bulgur.

PROVENÇAL LUNCH

SERVES TWO LUNCHBOXES

Chicken rustic roll

- *1 baguette*
- *1 tablespoon mayonnaise*
- *a handful of pitted black olives, sliced*
- *60g cooked and shredded chicken*
- *1 tomato, roasted*
- *1 red pepper, roasted*
- *1 large mushroom, roasted*
- *1 teaspoon pesto*
- *olive oil*

Easy homemade pesto

- *2 tablespoons mixed pumpkin, sesame and sunflower seeds*
- *1 cup packed fresh basil*
- *juice of 1 lemon*
- *¼ cup olive oil to start (add if necessary)*

Blend all the pesto ingredients until smooth. Add oil if necessary. Pour over the vegetable salad and stir until all the ingredients are evenly combined.

Homemade mayonnaise

- *1 egg*
- *salt and coarse-ground black pepper*
- *1 teaspoon mustard powder*
- *2 tablespoons white wine vinegar*
- *350ml oil (more may be added for a thicker consistency)*

Condiments

- *2 hard-boiled eggs*
- *1 avocado, peeled, deboned and sliced lengthwise*
- *Greek yoghurt drizzled with honey*
- *a handful of raspberries*

Chocolate brownie

- *225g unsalted butter*
- *300g dark chocolate chips*
- *½ teaspoon vanilla extract*
- *275g castor sugar*
- *135g plain flour*
- *¼ teaspoon salt*

Chicken rustic roll

Roast the red pepper, tomato and mushroom in a baking tray. In a small bowl, mix the olive oil and pesto, then stir and pour over the vegetables. Roast in a preheated oven at 200 for about 15 minutes. Set aside to cool.

Halve the baguette lengthwise. Spread the mayonnaise, place the chicken and olives over the bottom half of the roll, and arrange the vegetables evenly. Close the topping with the other half of the bread and press firmly while portioning the bread in quarters.

Homemade mayonnaise

Put the egg into a bowl of a fruit processer with the rest of the ingredients except for the oil. While blending, add the oil in a slow and steady stream. The colour should change from yellow to pale, to almost white, and the mayonnaise begins to thicken. Check the seasoning and the consistency, adding more salt and more vinegar if necessary. Pour in a sterilised glass jar and store in a refrigerator for up to a week.

Chocolate brownie

Preheat the oven at 160 and grease a square 23 cm baking tray. Melt the butter and ⅔ of the chocolate chips in a saucepan over low heat. Do not let the mixture become too warm. Whisk the eggs, vanilla and sugar. When the butter mixture is cool, add it to the eggs and sugar. Beat until smooth, then add the sifted flour. Keep mixing till everything is completely combined. Fold the remaining chocolate chips until evenly distributed. Pour into the prepared baking dish and bake for 20 minutes until the top is set and firm but inside still soft and gooey. Cut in squares after the brownies have cooled completely.

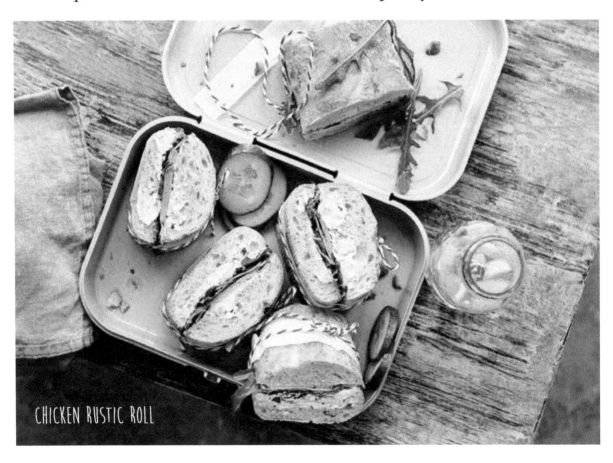

CHICKEN RUSTIC ROLL

FOOD ACCORDING TO LOCAL TRADITIONS

SPAIN

Spain is a country in the western Mediterranean basin. Together with Portugal, it forms part of the Iberian Peninsula. It is situated to the north of the British Overseas Territory of Gibraltar. The people of Spain are called Spaniards. Spanish is the national language, while other languages include Eustaki, Andalusian, Valenciano, Galician and Catalan. The religion of most of the people in Spain is Roman Catholic.

Since 1975, Spain has had a king, but daily political business is run by the government. For example, the king can declare a war but only if the government asks him to do so. Parliament, called "Las Cortes Generales", has two levels, the Congress and the Senate, and it is chosen by the Spanish people through General Elections. The government and the king's palace are in Madrid, the country's capital.

Spain has more than 500,000 square kilometres of land. It is smaller than France, but bigger than Sweden or Italy. Almost sixty million people live in Spain.

Spain is famous for its scenery which includes many UNESCO recognised heritage sites like the Gaudí architecture, Moorish quarters, sixteenth-century fortresses, and decorated caves. In addition, Spain houses the well-preserved artworks in history dating to the fifteenth century and earlier.

Spain is also known for its culinary delights which include the most famous tapas culture with different kinds of cheeses, olives, chorizo sausages, prawns, crackers, potatoes, and ham served for every meal. Introduced as something to nibble until dinner time, the tapas culture evolved into a food ritual that amazes people worldwide. The small portion of snacks include some of the most famous Spanish dishes, that is to say jamón ibérico (Iberian ham), squid, Spanish omelettes, patatas bravas, marinated olives, and mouth-watering cheeses.

MEXICO

Mexico is a land of extremes, with high mountains and deep canyons in the centre of the country, sweeping deserts in the north, and dense rain forests in the south and east.

Mexico is the product of a rich Native American heritage, three centuries of Spanish rule, and a shared border with the world's richest country, the United States. Today, many Mexicans are "mestizos" which means they have a mix of Native American and Spanish blood.

Throughout its history, Mexico has been home to great artists. The Maya and other Native Americans made impressive murals, sculptures, and jewellery. Modern Mexican artists include great painters, photographers, sculptors and muralists. Magdalena Carmen Frida Kahlo y Calderón, known worldwide as Frida Kahlo, a painter known for her many portraits and self-portraits, is just one of them.

Mexico is rich in natural resources like oil, silver, copper, and agricultural products. Its economy boasts a rich diversity of agricultural crops, highly productive oil fields and a growing manufacturing base. Contrary to popular belief, bullfighting and rodeo were invented in Mexico.

The origins of Mexican cuisine may be traced back to the Mayan civilisation that firmly believed that the richness of food could enrich the spirit and the body of a person through various sensory perceptions like taste, smell and touch. Traditional Mexican meals include a wide use of chocolates, peanuts, tomatoes, beans and vanilla, combined with cheese, pork, beef and lamb. These meat delicacies are perfectly complemented by land-grown vegetables, corn, tropical fruits and beans. Corn is widely considered a basic supplement in Mexican dishes as it is widely grown and was therefore an integral part of the country's culture.

VIETNAM

Vietnam is a long, narrow nation shaped like the letter S. It is in southeast Asia, on the eastern edge of the peninsula known as Indochina. Its neighbours include China to the north, and Laos and Cambodia to the west. At its narrowest point, Vietnam is only 48 kilometres wide. Two of Vietnam's largest rivers, the Mekong in the south and the Red in the north, end at the South China Sea in huge swampy plains called deltas. These regions are home to most of the country's people and provide fertile ground for the growing of rice and many other crops.

Most Vietnamese people live in the countryside, mainly in the river delta regions of the north and south. Recently though, people have begun to move to the main cities of Hồ Chí Minh, formerly Saigon, and Hanoi.

As a communist country, Vietnam has no official religion. But people are free to worship if they want to, and many follow what is called the "Three Teachings" of Confucianism, Taoism, and Buddhism.

Vietnam was ruled by the Hung kings as from the third century BC. Chinese troops invaded the northern parts of the country in 111 BC and then various Chinese dynasties ruled the area. In the eighteenth century, the peninsula was colonised by France and from 1858 until 1954 the country formed part of French Indochina. After the end of the Second World War and the declaration of independence in 1945, the French continued to rule the country until 1954. Then Vietnam was divided into North Vietnam and South Vietnam, and the country was shocked by the violent Second Indonesian War from 1955 to 1975. This war is also referred to as the "Resistance War Against America" or the "American War". Saigon fell on 30 April 1975, and the city was subsequently renamed Hồ Chí Minh City in honour of the fallen Vietnamese communist leader Hồ Chí Minh.

The main agricultural products are rice, coffee, tea and pepper as well as soybeans, cashews and peanuts. Vietnamese food is a blend of Chinese and Thai styles, and features seafood and homegrown fruits and vegetables. Many dishes in Vietnam consist mainly of rice, vegetables, fish, seafood, chicken and beef. Soy sauce, fish sauce or shrimp sauce are the most common ingredients in Vietnamese dishes. The most popular way of cooking these ingredients in Vietnam is by stir-frying on very high heat.

THE PERSIAN EMPIRE

The Persian Empire was one of the greatest empires in ancient history, controlling an area greater than any other civilisation stretching from Anatolia, now part of Turkey, and Egypt across to the north of India and Central Asia. It lasted from 550 to 330 BC.

Like most great empires in history, Persia started small. Kings ruled Persia, today's Iran, for many years. However, a kingdom only becomes an empire when it begins to take over its neighbours. The first Persian king to do so, Cyrus II, conquered neighbouring Turkey in 550 BC, eventually overpowering the whole middle east region.

While Cyrus laid the borders of the Persian Empire, it was another emperor named Darius who made Persia prosperous. Darius built roads throughout the empire for communication and trade, and created the system of governors called "satraps" who would rule the various provinces. Darius also conquered the northern part of India, thereafter building a new capital city called Persepolis. He went on to be remembered as Darius the Great.

The most important period of the Persian Empire came during a long series of wars with Greece. The Persians controlled next-door Turkey, but many people living there considered themselves Greeks and rebelled against Persia. These Greeks were supported by powerful cities like Athens and Sparta.

In the end, the satraps became less loyal to the emperor and showed signs that they too wanted more freedom and power. They started supporting a young Macedonian king and military leader who was to become known worldwide as Alexander the Great. The latter began his conquest of the Persian Empire in 334 BC. He took over all the former Persian provinces and reached as far as India.

ITALY

Italy is a country in southern Europe. It is a democratic republic and is a founding member of the European Union. The Italian flag is green, white and red. The country has influenced the cultural and social development of the whole Mediterranean area.

Before 1861, it was made up of smaller kingdoms, principalities and city states. Italy has become famous for its wine, landscape, historical and artistic sites as well as its food that varies between regions.

The country's capital, Rome, is one of the most famous cities in the world, as it was the capital of the Roman Empire. Other famous cities in Italy include Venice, Naples, Genoa, Florence, Palermo and Milan.

In Italy, people enjoy leisurely meals, taking time for cooking, eating and telling stories when sharing food with family and friends. Some of the most popular Italian dishes include pizza, tagliatelle alla Bolognese, lasagne, gelato, polenta, pesto, mozzarella, parmeggiano-reggiano cheese, Parma ham, grissini and tiramisù.

TUSCANY

Tuscany (Toscana in Italian) is a region in central Italy. It has an area of 22,990 km^2 and a population of about four million people. The capital city is Florence. Tuscany is known for its landscapes and its artistic legacy.

Six Tuscan localities have been made UNESCO protected sites, namely the historical centre of Florence, the historical core of Siena, the square of the Cathedral in Pisa, the main piazza of San Gimignano, the historical centre of Pienza and the Val d'Orcia.

Tuscany is known for its wines including the most famous chianti, Vino Nobile di Montepulciano and Brunello di Montalcino. It has 120 protected regional nature reserves that are used to help produce agricultural products including Chianina cattle famous as the "Fiorentina" steak and the production of olive oil.

TUSCAN FROLLINI BISCUITS

The history of these Tuscan biscuits takes us back to medieval times, to the time of conflict between the political rivals Ghibellines and Guelphs and the battle of Campaldino. After the latter battle, the Guelph party split into two separate parties named the White Guelphs and the Black Guelphs. The Tuscan frollini have been made for generations with flour or chocolate powder, thereby representing the colours of the White Guelphs and the Black Guelphs.

The famous Italian poet Dante Alighieri supported the White Guelphs who supported a greater degree of freedom from Rome. In 1301, the Pope backed the Black Guelphs who took over the city of Florence and plundered it. Dante was sent in exile and was fined heavily. Later in his life he supported several attempts by the White Guelphs to retake Florence, but all of those attempts failed.

DANTE ALIGHIERI

Dante Alighieri lived during the late medieval period. His original work "Divine Comedy" is considered an all-time classic in the Italian language. He is credited with establishing the national language of Italy. His style inspired famous minds like John Milton, William Shakespeare and Alfred Lord Tennyson.

Dante was born in 1265 in Florence. His family was heavily involved in politics. The poet was greatly influenced politically by his father Alighiero di Bellincione who supported the Guelph party in its struggle against the Holy Roman Emperor. Dante later became a pharmacist to further his political career. Although Dante held several public offices, his political career did not take off the way he desired.

According to a custom of that period, Dante was betrothed at the age of twelve to a girl from a rich and influential family. However he had fallen in love with a girl named Beatrice. His love for Beatrice inspired him to write "Vita Nuova". Dante eventually ended up marrying his fiancée, Gemma.

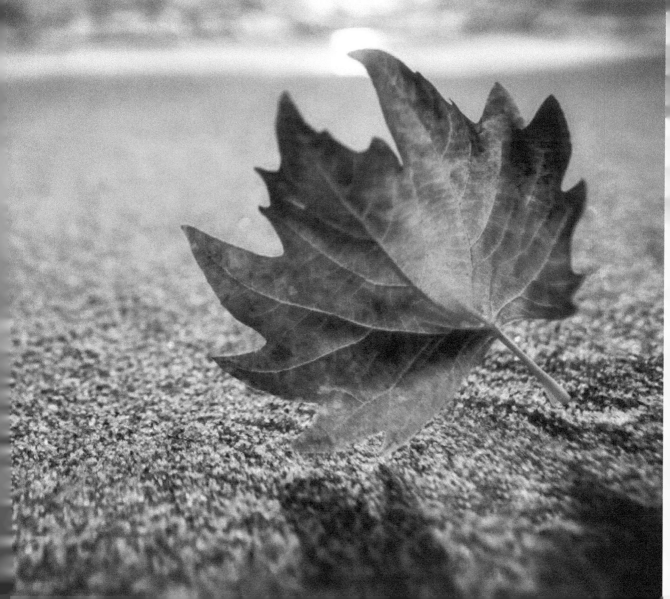

GRAND FINALE
LUNCHBOX

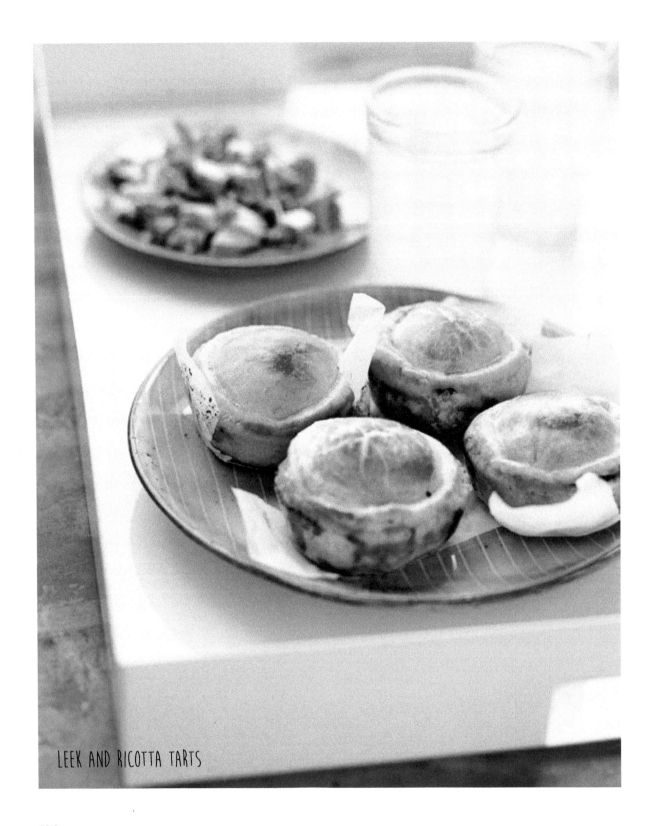

LEEK AND RICOTTA TARTS

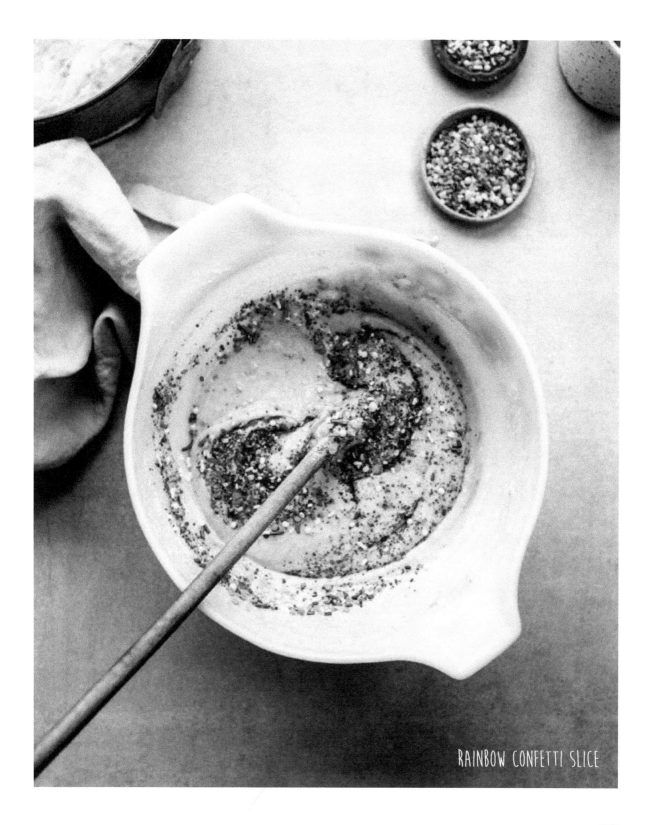

RAINBOW CONFETTI SLICE

LEEK AND RICOTTA TARTS
***
RAINBOW CONFETTI SLICE

SERVES TWO LUNCHBOXES

Leek and ricotta tarts

- 500g ricotta
- ¼ cup parmesan, grated
- 2 eggs
- 600g ready-prepared shortcrust pastry
- 1 leek, finely sliced
- 40g butter
- 2 teaspoons thyme

Mediterranean salad

- 60g feta cheese, cut in cubes
- a handful of kalamata olives
- 1 tomato, cut in chunks
- 2 artichoke hearts, halved, or ½ a cucumber cut in chunks
- 1 teaspoon dried oregano

Mix all the ingredients together with a dash of olive oil.

Rainbow confetti slice

- 1 cup unsalted butter, room temperature
- ⅓ cup vegetable oil
- 1¾ cups sugar
- 3 large eggs, room temperature
- 3 large egg whites, room temperature
- 1 tablespoon vanilla extract
- 3 cups all-purpose flour
- 2 teaspoons baking powder
- 1 teaspoon salt
- 1 cup Greek yoghurt, room temperature
- ¼ cup rainbow sprinkles

Condiments

- 2 tubs organic small strawberry yoghurts
- 2 whole clementines
- 4 soft dates
- a handful of dried apple slices

Leek and ricotta tarts

Pre-heat the oven to 180°C. Place ricotta, eggs and parmesan in a bowl and whisk until smooth. In a pan, cook some butter over medium heat and sautée the leeks and thyme until softened. When cooled, add them to the ricotta mixture and stir until all the ingredients are evenly combined.

Roll out the pastry over a floured surface and place over a baking pie tray lined with parchment paper. Alternatively line a 9-hole muffin tray and make individual pies. Fill the pastry with spoonfuls of ricotta mixture and season well with salt and pepper. Cover the filling with another layer of pastry and brush with melted butter or egg wash. Bake for 25-30 minutes until golden.

Rainbow confetti slice

Pre-heat oven to 180°C. Grease a small baking cake dish and line with parchment paper. In a large bowl, cream the butter, oil and sugar for 5-7 minutes until light and fluffy. Add eggs, then egg whites, one at a time, beating well after each addition. Finally, add the vanilla. In another bowl, whisk flour, baking powder and salt, and add to the creamed mixture alternately with the Greek yoghurt, beating well after each addition. Fold in the sprinkles.

Transfer to the prepared pan. Bake for 35-40 minutes until golden, risen and a toothpick inserted in centre comes out clean. Cool completely on a wire rack.

CONCLUSION

Preparing school lunches can become rather tedious. This book is designed to help parents inspire their children to explore different foods from around the world. Adding colour and flavour to daily lunches can add nutrients and ensure variety. This manual has been designed to arouse the curiosity of children by (i) exposing the provenance of certain food items, (ii) relating some interesting facts concerning the countries those items come from, (iii) describing fun facts related to some food items, and (iv) commemorating some historical moments pertaining to the different foods. It is hoped that the interconnection between the recipes and the fun facts narrated in this book will encourage children to be more adventurous with their food and make healthier choices. We envisage parents cooking while listening to fun facts narrated by their children, creating special moments that may be relived through the lunchboxes prepared.

Kids love lunch-times at school. Opening a lunchbox filled with delicious snacks that mum or dad would have packed for them can give them an enormously positive boost to the day. Packing a healthy, attractive and varied lunchbox for your kids is an expression of love. The key is to provide food that is easy for them to eat, and to provide it in lunchboxes that are easy for them to open. Bento boxes in Japan are hailed as something meant to show affection. They are indeed considered an act of love.

School lunches should have a balance of food groups. They should include vegetables, fruit, carbohydrates, proteins and healthy fats to boost nutrition and make sure the kids are getting their essential vitamins and minerals ensuring a healthy and balanced lunch. Plan ahead dinner and the following day's lunch at the same time so as to utilise leftovers as part of the lunchbox. This way, you will save time in the morning rush. Freeze all your baking, portioned, and utilise when needed. It is a great way to have treats available at any given time.

If school mornings are too rushed, consider packing the lunches the night before. Making a lunchbox while preparing dinner provides enough time to make a balanced and healthy lunchbox. Meals prepared from scratch usually contain more nutrients, fewer calories, chemicals and sweeteners than pre-packaged foods. Get the kids involved. Cooking creates a sense of ownership that shifts their perception and relationship with food. Teaching children to cook not only educates them about nutrition, it also teaches them to make smarter food choices and take a greater care in planning.

Time spent cooking with children when they are still young offers a relaxed opportunity to communicate. Involving children and youngsters in the process of lunchbox-making can expand major components of communication which include listening, talking and reading. It is an investment that will pay off as children grow. The time that you spend together in the kitchen while chatting and cooking becomes even more important as children reach the adolescent and teenage years.

Family habits established during the early years will carry through to the young adult years. A healthy love of cooking, and experience in the kitchen is an essential life skill that will lead to success when children move from home to live independently, or when they find themselves in relationships with shared responsibilities.

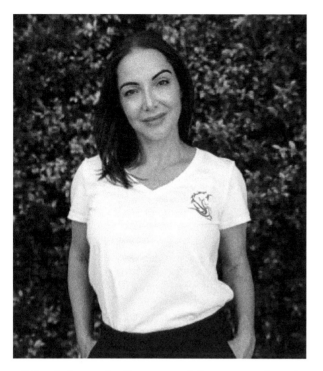

AUDREY SCHAERRER'S PROFILE

Audrey Schaerrer attended the American College of Sports Medicine (ACSM) in Indianapolis, United States of America, and qualified in Fitness Management, Nutritional Therapy and Science of Exercise. She has been practising as a nutritional therapist and food specialist in Europe for over twenty years.

Audrey is mother to an 11-year-old girl, and she considers motherhood as an exciting living experience. She has always affirmed and demonstrated that raising children constitutes a passion which no mother should set aside, and that strongly positive values should be imbued in one's own children for them to grow up as true and genuine leaders of tomorrow's world. This publication highlights the importance of children's attendance in the kitchen where they may watch and partake in the preparation of their family's eating patterns.

Audrey's mission is (i) to help busy parents and individuals lead a healthier lifestyle with fuss-free, varied, delicious meal plans and products, (ii) to introduce delicious foods that enhance physical and mental health, as well as general wellbeing, and (iii) to help clients look after their health naturally, lowering cholesterol, controlling blood pressure, and properly tackling functional gastrointestinal disorders by means of a naturally healthier lifestyle. Audrey's view is that, like medicine, food can help avoid many illnesses in adults and children including diabetes, high blood pressure, high cholesterol, depression, cancer and heart-related illnesses.

Her core belief in raising children through example has driven her to create a platform which is accessible to all persons who wish to enjoy a healthier lifestyle and who are eager to see healthy nutrition becoming a target at everybody's reach.

Lightning Source UK Ltd.
Milton Keynes UK
UKHW050610091022
410078UK00005B/36